ALLE ZEIT WACH
1842

B. Scharrer E.M. Smith G.B. Stefano
(Eds.)

Neuropeptides and Immunoregulation

With 19 Figures and 13 Tables

Springer-Verlag
Berlin Heidelberg New York
London Paris Tokyo
Hong Kong Barcelona
Budapest

Dr. Berta Scharrer
Albert Einstein College of Medicine
Dept. of Anatomy and Structural Biology
1300 Morris Park Avenue
Bronx, NY 10461-1736, USA

Dr. Eric M. Smith
University of Texas Medical Branch
Dept. of Psychiatry and Behavioral Sciences
Galveston, TX 77550, USA

Dr. George B. Stefano
Neuroscience Institute
State University of New York
College at Old Westbury
Old Westbury, NY 11568, USA

ISBN 3-540-57188-4 Springer-Verlag Berlin Heidelberg New York
ISBN 0-387-57188-4 Springer-Verlag New York Berlin Heidelberg

Library of Congress Cataloging-in-Publication Data. Neuropeptides and immunoregulation / B. Scharrer, E. Smith, G.B. Stefano (eds.). p. cm. Includes bibliographical references and index. ISBN 0-387-57188-4 (New York). – ISBN 3-540-57188-4 (Berlin) 1. Neuropeptides – Immunology. 2. Immune response – Regulation. 3. Cellular immunity. 4. Neuroimmunology. I. Scharrer, Berta, 1906– . II. Smith, E. (Eric) III. Stefano, George B., 1945– . QP552.N39N4855 1993 591.2′9 – dc20 93-32233

Printed in Germany

Typesetting: Thomson Press (I) Ltd., New Delhi

25/3130/SPS – 5 4 3 2 1 0 – Printed on acid-free paper

Preface

In the rapidly developing area of neuroimmunology, primary attention has been given thus far to the bidirectional exchange of information between the immune system and the neuroendocrine system. Several recent texts on this subject are based almost exclusively on experimental and clinical data obtained in mammalian species. One of the interesting insights gained from these studies is that the chemical messenger substances used in this exchange by either system are the same, or at least closely related to each other. Cytokines, primarily thought of as being dispatched by cells of the immune system, have recently been identified to be products of neural, in particular, glial elements. Conversely, neuropeptides formerly considered to be characteristic of the neuroendocrine apparatus are now known to be manufactured and dispatched by immunoregulatory cells as well.

The present text is the first to provide an overview of the rich body of information obtained in a series of broadly based comparative studies. This work in representatives of higher invertebrates has opened new vistas, in particular, regarding the immunomodulatory role played by opioid and other neuropeptides as signal molecules in the cell-mediated internal regulation of the immune system.

The remarkable parallels observed in the study of these phenomena in the two groups of animals have established certain general principles of neuro-immunobiological integration that have basic biological as well as biomedical implications. These commonalities, which are addressed in several chapters of this volume, can be summarized as follows. A number of neuropeptides have been demonstrated to act in an immunoregulatory capacity. Depending on their concentration and other factors, they may enhance or depress the activation of immunocompetent cells, a process judged by characteristic changes in cellular conformation. In all forms studied thus far, these modulatory activities are mediated by highly specific receptors. The opioid neuropeptide Met-enkephalin has been found to play a special role in immunoregulation, in contradistinction to the closely related Leu-enkephalin. This distinction does not apply to the roles played by these two substances in the nervous system. Another general feature is that the efficacy of certain neuropeptides, in their neuroimmunomodulatory capacity, is down-regulated by special enzymatic action, i.e., that of neutral endopeptidase 24.11. The use of a specific enzyme inhibitor (phosphoramidon) in slide tests has been shown to enhance the potency of Met-enkephalin in invertebrates as well as in vertebrates. In both groups, the effect of adrenocorticotropin on immune responses appears to be at least in part indirect, namely by giving rise to α-melanotropin, with which it shares its immunosuppressive effect. In invertebrates, coping with stressful stimuli, comparable to that in mammals, appears to engage the participation of neuropeptides of central nervous system origin. Furthermore, the interplay of neuropeptides with certain cytokines in invertebrates follows a pattern similar to that previously established in higher vertebrates.

Some of these common features explain certain clinical phenomena, such as the capacity of an invertebrate parasite (*Schistosoma*) to influence the immune response of a vertebrate host by releasing vertebrate-type immunosuppressive neuropeptides.

Bronx, NY, USA
Galveston, TX, USA
Old Westbury, NY, USA
January, 1994

BERTA SCHARRER
ERIC M. SMITH
GEORGE B. STEFANO

Contents

List of Contributors

Dr. ROBERT ADER
Departments of Psychiatry and Microbiology and Immunology
University of Rochester Medical Center, 601 Elmwood Avenue, Rochester, NY 14642, USA

Dr. J. EDWIN BLALOCK
Department of Physiology and Biophysics, University of Alabama at Birmingham, UAB Station, Birmingham, AL 35294-0001, USA

Dr. ROBERT CHIN
Department of Microbiology, J-19, University of Texas Medical Branch, Galveston, TX 77550, USA

Dr. NICHOLAS COHEN
Departments of Psychiatry and Microbiology and Immunology
University of Rochester Medical Center, 601 Elmwood Avenue, Rochester, NY 14642, USA

Dr. DEBORAH V. HARBOUR
Department of Human Biological Chemistry and Genetics and Microbiology, University of Texas, Medical Branch, Galveston, TX 77550, USA

Dr. THOMAS K. HUGHES
Department of Microbiology, J-19, University of Texas Medical Branch, Galveston, TX 77550, USA

Dr. BRANISLAV D. JANKOVIĆ
Immunology Research Center, Vojvode Stepe 458, Belgrade, Yugoslavia

Dr. MICHAEL K. LEUNG
Department of Chemistry, State University of New York College at Old Westbury, Old Westbury, NY 11568-0210, USA

Dr. DRAGAN MARIĆ
Immunology Research Center, Vojvode Stepe 458, Belgrade, Yugoslavia

Dr. JAN E. MOYNIHAN
Departments of Psychiatry and Microbiology and Immunology University of Rochester Medical Center, 601 Elmwood Avenue, Rochester, NY 14642, USA

Dr. BERTA SCHARRER
Department of Anatomy and Structural Biology, Albert Einstein College of Medicine, 1300 Morris Park Avenue, Bronx, NY 10461-1736, USA

Dr. ERIC M. SMITH
Department of Psychiatry and Behavioral Sciences, University of Texas Medical Branch, Galveston, TX 77550, USA

Dr. GEORGE B. STEFANO
Old Westbury Neuroscience Research Institute, State University of New York College at Old Westbury, Old Westbury, NY 11568-0210, USA

Dr. ANTHONY J. TURNER
Department of Biochemistry and Molecular Biology, The University of Leeds, Leeds, LS2 9JT, UK

Dr. DENNIS VAN EPPS
Baxter Health Care Corporation, Applied Sciences, WG2-2S, Baxter Technology Park, Round Lake, IL 60073, USA

Dr. DOUGLAS A. WEIGENT
Department of Physiology and Biophysics, University of Alabama at Birmingham, UAB Station, Birmingham, AL 35294-0001, USA

Neuropeptides and Autoregulatory Immune Processes

B. Scharrer[1] and G. B. Stefano[2]

Introduction

Bioactive neuropeptides, formerly thought of primarily as signal molecules confined to the nervous system, are now known to be widely distributed in the organism. One of the multiple roles of these messenger substances is their participation in the coordination of internal immunoregulatory processes (van Epps and Saland 1984; Fischer and Falke 1984). Most of the vertebrate data referred to in this and several other chapters have been obtained from mammalian studies. In recent years a rich body of information has been added to these observations based on the use of representatives of two invertebrate phyla, molluscs and insects.

A major new insight gained in this area is that, in invertebrates as well as vertebrates, the substances involved in chemical communication among immunoactive cells are the same, or closely related to those used in the bidirectional exchange of information between the immune system and the neuroendocrine apparatus (Blalock 1989; Weigent and Blalock, this volume). There is ample evidence demonstrating that immunoregulatory processes can be enhanced as well as suppressed by this family of compounds, especially by opioid peptides. The substances acting in this capacity are produced and dispatched by immunoactive cells which respond to their presence in a receptor-mediated fashion. It is particularly in the area of autoimmunoregulation that recent results obtained in invertebrates have revealed remarkable parallels with those based on vertebrate studies.

Modulation of Cell-Mediated Autoregulatory Immune Processes

Two activities associated with immunoinflammatory reactions that have been analyzed in some detail in representatives of higher invertebrates as well as vertebrates are cellular adherence and locomotory activity of immunocompetent

[1] Department of Anatomy and Structural Biology, Albert Einstein College of Medicine, Bronx, NY 10461–1736, USA
[2] Old Westbury Neuroscience Research Institute, State University of New York at Old Westbury, Old Westbury, NY 11568–0210, USA

Scharrer et al. (Eds.)
Neuropeptides and Immunoregulation

cells. In the mollusc *Mytilus edulis* and the insect *Leucophaea maderae* these processes have been shown to be modulated by neuropeptides in the same way as in mammalian species (see Janković and Marić, this volume). Many of the respective in vitro and in vivo experiments have been carried out with various exogenous neuropeptides, for example, a stable synthetic analog of Met-enkephalin, D-Ala^2-Met^5-enkephalin, or enkephalinamide; (DAMA). Human neutrophils were also exposed to Met-enkephalin, substance P, and the synthetic tripeptide *N*-formyl-methionyl-leucyl-phenylalanine (f-MLP). In addition, the effects of endogenous opioids, isolated from the hemolymph of *Mytilus*, were examined (Stefano et al. 1989b).

In vertebrates the classification of mononuclear and polymorphonuclear cell types specializing in these and other functions of the immune system is well established. A number of in vitro experiments were carried out with populations of granulocytes or T-lymphocytes from mammalian blood (Stefano et al. 1989b; Heagy et al. 1990; Shipp et al. 1990).

The immunoactive invertebrate cells, responding to opioid and additional messenger substances in much the same way as their mammalian counterparts, are subpopulations of the animals' hemocytes. Ultrastructurally they are characterized by the presence of conspicuous cytoplasmic granules and other organelles resembling those of vertebrate granulocytes (see Scharrer 1972; Renwrantz 1990). In light of present knowledge, a classification of immunoactive hemocytes based on ultrastructural parameters is not yet possible. However, the premise that special hemocytes are active in immunoregulatory processes of invertebrates is supported by ample experimental evidence obtained primarily in *Mytilus* and *Leucophaea* (Stefano et al. 1989a,b) and recently in *Proptera alata* (Finn et al. 1991). These specialized invertebrate hemocytes are therefore referred to as immunocytes.

For in vitro studies preparations of invertebrate and vertebrate immunocytes were examined by phase contrast and Nomarski optics coupled with a Zeiss Axiophot Microscope. Measurements were taken with either the Zeiss Videoplan/Vidas Image Analysis System or that designed by American Innovision (San Diego, CA). Specific images were converted to binary images, following frame grabbing and before recordings were made. Cells were photographed by an internal Zeiss-Automated Program Photography System (35-mm film) and a timelapse video synchronization system (JVC).

Changes in cellular conformation, determined by measurements of cellular area and perimeter, were expressed mathematically by the form-factor-pe calculation of the Zeiss Vidas Analysis System, whereby the equation $4 \times \pi \times$ area/perimeter^2 provides mean numerical values. The lower this number, the higher is the cellular perimeter and the more ameboid the cellular shape. The velocity of cellular locomotion was determined by measuring the distance traveled over time.

The characterization of morphometric changes in stimulated immunocytes can be carried a step further by use of the image analysis system recently introduced by Schön et al. (1991). The addition of two factors (circular and elliptical) to the form-factor equation permits a distinction as to the type of cellular change. Circularity denotes an increase in cellular area and perimeter as a result of flattening, by which a cell remains relatively rounded. Elliptical change refers to the same phenomenon, i.e., increase in cell size, resulting in an elliptical shape.

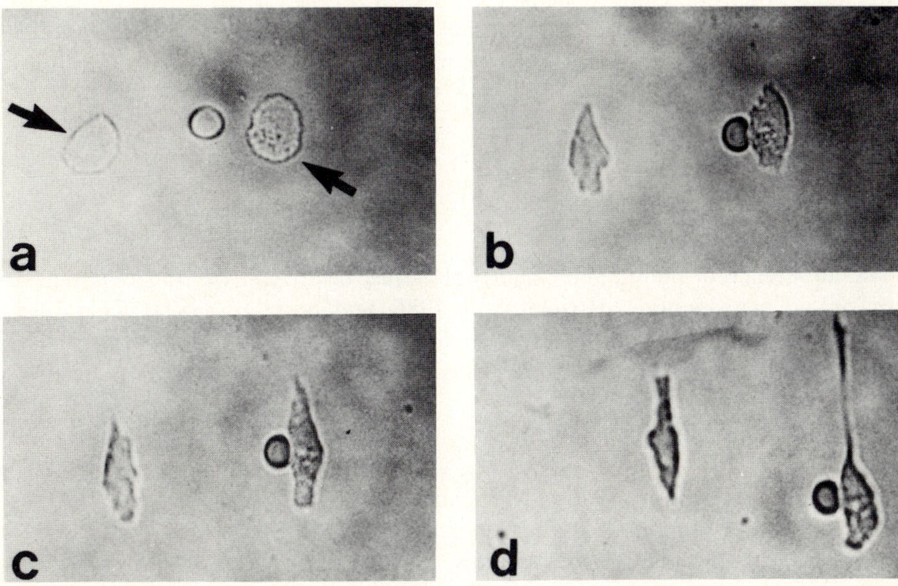

Fig. 1a–d. Stimulation of human leukocytes by DAMA (10^{-11} *M*). **a** Unstimulated cells (*arrows*) next to an erythrocyte. **b–d** Same cells exposed to opioid observed at intervals of 1·5, 3, and 4·5 min. Note gradual elongation. Means of form-factor-pe values: 0·81 (**a**) and 0·41 (**d**). (From Stefano et al. 1989b)

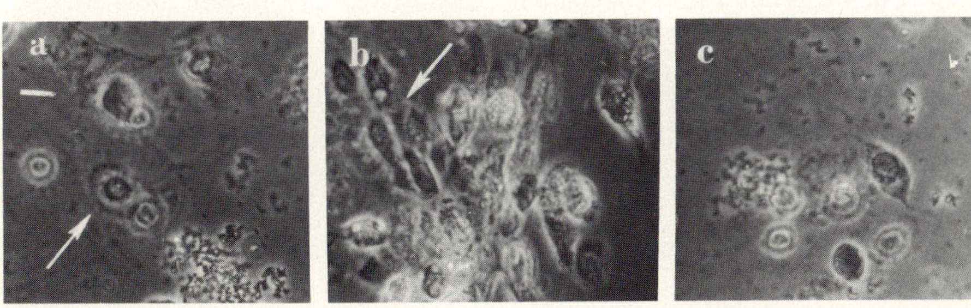

Fig. 2a–c. Immunocytes of *Leucophaea maderae*. **a** Prior to opioid stimulation; note rounded cells (*arrow*). **b** Thirty minutes after exposure to DAMA (10^{-11} *M*); note elongate activated cells (*arrow*). **c** Thirty minutes after exposure to both DAMA and naloxone (10^{-8} *M*); note blocking of activation of immunocytes. Means of form-factor values are 0·81 (**a**), 0·47 (**b**), and 0·79 (**c**). *Bar*, 10 μm. (From Stefano et al. 1989b)

Use of this new form-factor formula permits differentiation not only among responses obtained in different animal species to the same signal molecule, for example, elongation in human (Fig. 1b–d) and *Leucophaea* immunocytes (Fig. 2b) versus ameboid change in *Mytilus*, in the presence of one signal molecule such as DAMA, but also among the effects of different substances in the same species. For example, whereas DAMA was found to produce more or less ameboid shapes in activated immunocytes of *Mytilus*, lipopolysaccaride resulted in enlarged cells of rounded shape (Schön et al. 1991).

Mean values were based on 20 individual readings taken from different cells. Individual points on the graphs are the means of from three to five mean values. These final means did not vary by more than 6%.

Cellular Adherence

The adherence of mammalian neutrophils has been reported to be enhanced by opioid neuropeptides (Brown et al. 1986; Stefano et al. 1989a). This dose-dependent effect is bimodal, and its mediation by high-affinity receptors can be concluded indirectly from the observation that the high-affinity peak is counteracted by naloxone.

In human neutrophils, the synthetic tripeptide f-MLP (10^{-7}–10^{-12} *M*) and substance P (10^{-11} *M*) have been shown to modulate the expression of two cell-surface adhesion molecules, Mo 1 and LAM-1. Exposure to f-MLP causes upregulation of Mo 1 and downregulation of LAM-1 (Shipp et al. 1991).

Similarly, immunocytes of *Mytilus, Leucophaea*, and *Proptera* respond to low concentrations of opioids by adhering to albumin-coated slides and the formation of clumps (Stefano et al. 1989a; Finn et al. 1991). DAMA produces this effect in a concentration of 10^{-11} *M*, and naloxone (10^{-8} *M*,) blocks it, in a dose-response manner. Tests carried out with naloxone revealed that, depending on its concentration, it may act either as an agonist or an antagonist. By contrast, exogenous Met-enkephalin administered in the same low dose as DAMA does not enhance cellular adherence. This difference in potency is due to the presence of a special proteolytic enzyme (enkephalinase, neutral endopeptidase 24.11) in the hemolymph, which affects DAMA to a much smaller degree than Met-enkephalin (see below, and Turner et al., this volume).

Migratory Behavior of Immunocytes

Vertebrates

An important functional property of polymorphonuclear leukocytes (PMN), lymphocytes, and monocytes is that in addition to random movements (chemokinesis) they show migratory behavior directed toward sites of inflammation or antigenic challenge (chemotaxis; Van Epps et al. 1983; Brown et al. 1986). Apparently they reach their destinations guided by concentration gradients of the signal substances involved.

Evidence supporting the concept that opioid peptides are involved in the chemotactic movement of mammalian immunocytes has been provided by several in vivo and in vitro studies. For example, chronic infusion of several opioids elicited directed migration of neutrophils, macrophages, and lymphocyte-type cells (Brown et al. 1986; Ruff and Pert 1986). The responsiveness of monocytes to opioids was found to be stronger than that of neutrophils. Moreover, immunocytes could be desensitized to certain opioids by prior exposure to them. Intraventricular injection of β-endorphin or Met-enkephalin resulted in the appearance of macrophagelike cells in the cerebrospinal fluid (Saland et al. 1983; Van Epps et al. 1983).

These opioid effects have been compared with the chemotactic activity of the synthetic peptide f-MLP. This substance stimulated a much larger proportion of immunocytes (80%) than the opioids tested (30%), and its effect was not blocked by naloxone. Furthermore f-MLP enhanced the migratory activity of neutrophils preexposed to β-endorphin (Simpkins et al. 1984).

According to Casale et al. (1984) opioids stimulate the release of inflammatory mediators (Janković and Marić, this volume). The question of the interaction of neuropeptides with other signal molecules, especially cytokines, in this activity is discussed by Hughes et al. (1990) and Hughes and Chin (this volume).

A recent in vitro study, carried out with a population of T-lymphocytes obtained from peripheral human blood (Heagy et al. 1990) clearly demonstrated that directed locomotion (chemotaxis) occurs in the presence of a concentration gradient of Met-enkephalin or β-endorphin, administered at concentrations of 10^{-11}–10^{-9} M. In the absence of such a gradient celluler movement was chemokinetic. Synthetic enkephalin analogs, including D-Ala^{2}-D-Leu^{5}-enkephalin (DADLE), D-Pen^{2}-D-Pen^{5}-enkephalin (DPDPE), and D-Ala^{2}-MePhe^{4}-Gly^{5}-enkephalin (DAGO), stimulated the T-cells to a lesser extent. The neuropeptide-induced chemotactic movements of T-cells are mediated by the interaction of ligands with binding sites analogous to opiate/opioid receptors (see Stefano, this volume).

Invertebrates

In vivo tests carried out in *Mytilus* showed that invertebrate immunocytes, like those of vertebrates, are capable of chemotactic movements brought about by concentration gradients of certain recognition factors (Stefano et al. 1989a). Severance of the branchial nerve evoked a cellular immune response, i.e., the recruitment and directed migration of activated cells to the lesioned area. The gradual increase in their quantity over a 10-h period could be readily monitored because *Mytilus* immunocytes are yellow-fluorescent due to the presence of serotonin.

Injections of DAMA into nonlesioned animals also resulted in directed movement and accumulation of immunocytes at the site of administration. The specificity of this opioid effect became apparent from the fact that it was blocked by naloxone, and that control injections of epinephrine, norepinephrine, dopamine, serotonin, insulin, octopamine, and FMRFamide (Phe-Met-Arg-Phe-amide) failed to elicit directed cellular movement to the site of injection (Stefano et al. 1989a).

The injection of DAMA placed in the vicinity of the severed nerve showed that after a period of 2-h the concentration gradient produced by the injected drug had taken precedence over that presumed to be provided by endogenous recognition factors dispatched at the site of lesion. This differential response may be explained in part by a critical difference in the concentrations of endogenous and injected ligands competing with each other for opioid receptors.

In vitro tests with the hemolymph of *Mytilus* and *Leucophaea* showed slight random movements in unstimulated immunocytes of these invertebrates. However, chemotactic movements and the formation of large cellular clumps occurred after the addition of opioid peptides to the incubation medium. In this case, single or small groups of immunocytes were seen to move toward larger accumulations of cells.

In summary, endogenous opioids, presumably in collaboration with cytokines and additional factors, play a role as signaling molecules in the recruitment of immunoactive cells (Kornfeld et al. 1985; Hughes and Chin, this volume).

Structural Signs and Time Course of Immunocyte Activation

Changes in the activity of immunocytes are preceded by characteristic conformational alterations (Figs. 1, 2). Prior to the onset of locomotory behavior, stimulated by opioid peptides, the following signs indicative of cellular activation are observed. Mammalian (Falke and Fischer 1986; Fischer and Falke 1986; Stefano 1989) and invertebrate cells (Stefano et al. 1989b), which in the inactive condition are more or less rounded, show an increase in cellular size and surface area and/or the formation of pseudopodia. For example, β-endorphin can induce mammalian PMNs to increase their diameter by approximately 20% in more than 30% of the total cell population examined. However, this phenomenon is not apparent in all vertebrate species tested thus far. It cannot be demonstrated in the rat and dog, but it is clearly noticeable in the rabbit (Falke and Fischer 1986) and very pronounced in man (Stefano et al. 1989b).

The addition of Met-enkephalin-Arg^{6}-Phe^{7} (10^{-9} M) to the incubation medium elicited conformational changes in approximately 37% of human and 32% of *Mytilus* granulocytes (Stefano et al. 1991a). These values are in the range of those previously reported for various other opioid substances (Stefano et al. 1989a, b). In both cell types examined the presence of DAMA (10^{-11} M) plus Met-enkephalin Arg^{6}-Phe^{7} in the incubation medium did not increase the proportion of responding cells (29%–33%). Therefore, the cell population activated by either opioid can be judged to be the same. As expressed by the

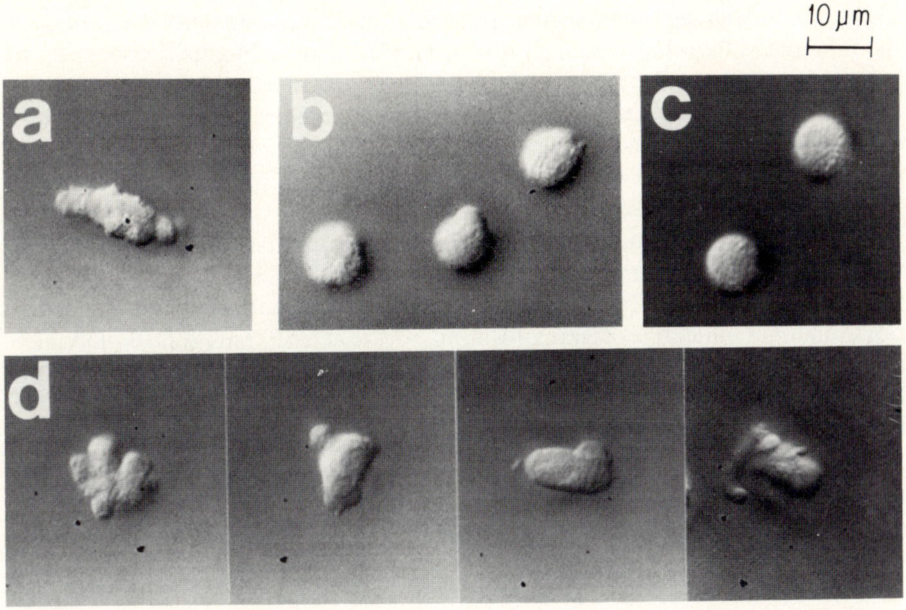

Fig. 3a–d. Enhancement of Met-enkephalin stimulation of human polymorphonuclear leukocytes by inhibition of CD10/NEP by special enzyme inhibitor phosphoramidon. Cells exposed to Met-enkephalin (10^{-6} *M*, **a**) Met-enkephalin (10^{-11} *M*, **b**) phosphoramidon (100 μ*M*, **c**), and Met-enkephalin (10^{-11} *M*) plus phosphoramidon (100 μ*M*, **d**)

form-factor analysis, the *Mytilus* cells responding to opioid stimulation appeared more ameboid (value below 0·4) than the human cells (value above 0·4). Human granulocytes tend to become rather elongated after stimulation (Figs. 1, 3), as do those of the insect *Leucophaea* (Fig. 2). It should be mentioned that in vertebrates and invertebrates some conformational changes may be observed in unstimulated cell preparations, but at a much lower frequency.

Human and invertebrate immunocytes show a significant difference with regard to the time course of their response to opioid stimulation. In the presence of Met-enkephalin-Arg^6-Phe^7 activation becomes most noticeable within a period of 15–45 min, in *Mytilus* preparations, and within 5–15 min in human cells (Stefano et al. 1991a). The latter also show a higher velocity (5 μm/min) as compared with that of the corresponding invertebrate cells (2·1 μm/min). The distances traveled by unstimulated control cells are lower, i.e., 2·1 μm/min and 0·9 μm/min, respectively.

Spectrum of Immunoactive Neuropeptides

Tests with exogenous neuropeptides and synthetic analogs in vertebrates and invertebrates have revealed a spectrum of substances with modulatory effects on certain immune processes (see Janković and Marić, this volume).

Endogeneous messenger molecules participating in autoregulatory activities of the immune system have been shown to be identical with or closely related to neuropeptides derived from neural tissue. More specifically, such peptides have been demonstrated in activated helper cells from human blood donors (Zurawski et al. 1986). Some of these cells express genes encoding for precursors of opioid peptides, i.e., proenkephalin and pro-opiomelanocortin (Smith and Blalock 1981; Lolait et al. 1984, 1986).

Endogenous immunoactive neuropeptide material (Met-enkephalin) has been identified also in immunocytes of the invertebrate *Mytilus edulis* (Stefano et al. 1989a). Ligands which, in addition to Met-enkephalin, elicited conformational changes indicative of changing immunocyte activity are DPDPE, DADLE and DAGO (Table 1). Among these, the Met-enkephalin analog DAMA and the heptapeptide Met-enkephalin-Arg^6-Phe^7 proved significantly more potent than the rest. The heptapeptide is a naturally occurring cleavage product of proenkephalin A which has been identified in nervous tissue of *Mytilus* (Leung and Stefano 1987). It has also been found in mammalian blood and is believed to be released from the pituitary and adrenal glands under conditions of sympathetic stress (Clement-Jones et al. 1980; Kimura et al. 1985).

Table 1. Effect of opioid and opiate compounds on immunocyte perimeter and area (modified from Stefano et al. 1989b)

Ligand	Cell perimenter change Effective concentration (10^{-N} *M*)	Cell area
Invertebrate		
Delta		
DAMA	11	11
DADLE	8	8
DPDPE	8	8
Deltorphin	11	11
Met-Enkephalin-Arg-Phe	10	10
MU		
DAGO	9	9
β-Casomorphin	9	9
Kappa		
Dynorphin	8	9
Bremazocine[a]	8	8
Ethylketo-cyclazocine	8	8
Epsilon (?)		
β-Endorphin	10	10
Human		
DAMA	11	11
DADLE	8	8
Deltorphin	11	11
Met-Enkephalin-Arg-Phe	10	10

DADLE, [D-Ala^2, D-Leu^5] enkephalin; DPDPE, [D-Pen^2, D-Pen^5] enkephalin; DAGO, [D-Ala^2, MePhe^4, Gly(ol)^5] enkephalin; β-casomorphin, H-Tyr-Pro-Phe-Pro-Gly-Pro-Ile-OH.
[a]Nonopioid substance. Modified from Stefano et al. 1989a.

DAMA proved most effective at a concentration as low as 10^{-11} *M*. DADLE, the compound most closely related to DAMA, had a potency (10^{-9} *M*) matching that of most other substances tested. It is of particular interest that DAMA proved equally potent in tests with human leukocytes (Table 1). The distinctly lower effectiveness of DADLE in both human and invertebrate immune reactions is in contrast to the situation in the mammalian nervous system where no discrepancy in the binding potency of Met-enkephalin and Leu-enkephalin has been observed (see Stefano, this volume).

Most of the opioid and nonopioid substances tested thus far stimulate the activity of immunocytes, but inhibitory effects have been recorded for adrenocorticotropic hormone (ACTH) and melanocyte-stimulating hormone (MSH) (see Smith, Van Epps, both this volume; Stefano et al. 1991b). Both of these peptides, derived from pro-opiomelanocortin, have been shown to inactivate immunocytes that are either spontaneously active or experimentally activated by other signal molecules. Spontaneously active polymorphonuclear leukocytes of man and immunocytes of *Mytilus* have been shown to return to the inactive state in the presence of ACTH and α-MSH in a dose-dependent manner (Stefano et al. 1991b; Smith et al. 1992). However, this effect is somewhat difficult to quantify since only 5%–10% of the harvested cells show the ameboid conformation indicative of apparently spontaneous activation. This effect became more evident when β-endorphin (10^{-10} *M*) was used to change the immunocytes of *Mytilus* from inactive to ameboid-active. The subsequent administration of α-MSH (10^{-5}–10^{-7} *M*) reversed this conformational change in over 20% of the total of 32% of β-endorphin stimulated cells (Stefano et al. 1991b). In another experiment, immunocytes of the same species previously activated by the cytokine tumor necrosis factor (TNF) became inactive following the administration of ACTH or α-MSH (Van Epps and Mason 1990; Stefano et al. 1991b). The activity and conformation of inactive immunocytes were unaffected by ACTH, α-MSH, and β-MSH. In tests examining possible effects of neuropeptides on the phagocytotic activity of immunocytes a stimulatory role of ACTH was observed in two molluscan species (Ottaviani et al. 1990; Stefano, unpublished).

Interaction of Multiple Regulatory Substances

Recognition of the remarkable parallels in the immunoregulatory roles played by neuropeptides in vertebrates and invertebrates led to a search among invertebrates for the presence of cytokines. As reported in greater detail by Hughes et al. 1990; and Hughes and Chin, this volume, the hemolymph of *Mytilus* was found to contain immunoactive interleukin (IL-1) as well as TNF-α. Its immunocytes responded to these molecules both in vitro and in vivo in a manner similar to that of human granulocytes. As in mammals, the effect of IL-1 on the autoregulatory process in this mollusc appears to be brought about at least in part indirectly, i.e., by its stimulatory effect on the formation of TNF. In short, more than one cytokine can be judged to participate in the operation of an effective network of signals in the immune system of invertebrates as well as vertebrates.

Mode of Operation of Diverse Immunomodulatory Substances in Autoregulatory Processes

The involvement of multiple regulatory substances and additional factors raises the question of how they interact and possibly compete with each other. The result seems to depend in part on the type or degree of challenge received by the immune system (See Janković and Marić, this volume). For example, the stimulation of immunocytes by opioids was found to reach a point where the cells no longer react to additional amounts of the drug or to the antagonistic effect of naloxone (Stefano et al. 1989b).

A point of particular interest is the existence of a mechanism controlling the degree of cellular activation by means of enzymatic degradation of a given signal molecule (see Shipp et al. 1990; Stefano et al. 1991a; Turner et al., this volume). This process of stabilization has been shown to operate in invertebrate as well as mammalian systems and is accomplished by a specific enzyme, neutral endopeptidase 24.11 (NEP; Fig. 3). This enzyme has been shown to downregulate, for example, the local concentration of Met-enkephalin and Met-enkephalin-Arg^6-Phe^7. Its effect can be counteracted by use of a potent and highly specific enzyme inhibitor, phosphoramidon, whose presence markedly potentiates the efficacy of both opioid ligands. Tests carried out with two major compounds resulting from the hydrolysis of Met-enkephalin-Arg^6-Phe^7 showed that they antagonize the effect of the heptapeptide, presumably by competing for part of the same receptor sites as those used by the agonist. The effective concentration of the tetrapeptide fragment Phe-Met-Arg-Phe was 10^{-7}–10^{-8} M and that of the tripeptide Tyr-Gly-Gly 10^{-6} M (Stefano et al. 1991a). Apparently, in the event of a rapidly initiated excessive immune response, a balancing mechanism is provided by the enzymatic generation of antagonistic fragments embedded in the agonist's molecule (van Ree et al. 1981).

It is of further interest that NEP is itself regulated by the degree of activation of an immunoactive cell (Shipp et al. 1991). Following the cell's stimulation by TNF, the activity of NEP is increased and consequently this cell's subsequent response to a neuropeptide, which serves as one of its substrates, is downregulated. This may be the mechanism responsible for the loss of responsiveness to repetitive opioid stimulation mentioned above. Moreover, NEP influences the process of immunosuppression in that it converts ACTH to MSH (Smith et al. 1992; Smith, this volume).

The biomedical importance of a well-balanced immunoregulatory system is illustrated by the consequence of interference with its normal operation. The role of neuropeptides in various forms of stress has been thoroughly explored (see Taché et al. 1989). Recent studies have shown that immunosuppression effected by neuropeptides may determine the course of certain diseases caused by parasites or viral infection. There is experimental evidence supporting the concept that in schistosomiasis the parasite escapes detection and an effective immune reaction in the host by using the same signal molecules operating in the human immune and autoimmunoregulatory system (Duvaux-Miret et al. 1992). The release of ACTH by the adult parasite, and its conversion to α-MSH by NEP on human PMNs, inactivates specific defense cells and thus interferes with proper surveillance. Furthermore, the human immunodeficiency virus appears to have the ability to stimulate the production of ACTH by human immune cells (Smith et al. 1992), thus creating a scenario similar to that described for the parasitic worm.

An additional point to be made is that the immunostimulatory effects of certain neuropeptides, for example ACTH and MSH, take place at lower concentrations (10^{-9}–10^{-12} *M*) than their immunosuppressive effects (around 10^{-8} *M*). Furthermore, a difference in effective concentrations can be observed with regard to immunostimulatory activities of two different neuropeptides, for example, β-endorphin (10^{-10} *M*) and Met-enkephalin (10^{-11} *M*). Since Met-enkephalin is readily degraded by NEP, and β-endorphin is relatively resistant to this enzyme, one may surmise that the effects of β-endorphin are more prolonged than those of Met-enkephalin.

Conclusions

In summary, autoimmunoregulation is a well-balanced process accomplished by a diversity of cell types making use of a number of signal molecules, including neuropeptides and their respective receptors. Several of these complex regulatory phenomena known in the mammalian system have counterparts in higher invertebrates. In both groups the proportion of cells that have the potential to respond to specific signals is relatively small. The speed of the response to an activating stimulus is influenced by previous stimulation of the reactive cells.

Neuropeptides, cytokines, and specific immunomodulatory enzymes have been well conserved in the course of evolution. In recent reviews Stefano (1986, 1988, 1991) has proposed that the stereoselective nature of the signal molecules and their receptors may well be the evolutionary force at work. The components of this system, including its synthesizing enzymes, had to evolve simultaneously in order for it to be operational.

Acknowledgements. The authors wish to thanks their collaborators in various projects outlined in this chapter. During the preparation of the manuscript the authors were partially supported by NIDA 47392, ADAMHA-MARC MH 17138, NSF INT-8803664, NIMH-NIDA-COR (G.B.S.) and NIH NS 22344 (B.S.) and State University of New York Research Foundation.

References

Blalock JE (1989) A molecular basis for bidirectional communication between the immune and neuroendocrine systems. Physiol Rev 69:1–32

Brown SL, Tokuda S, Saland LC, Van Epps DE (1986) Opioid peptides: effects on leukocyte migration. In: Plotnikoff NP, Faith RE, Murgo AJ, Good R (eds) Enkephalins and endorphins, stress and the immune system. Plenum, New York, pp 367–386

Casale TB, Bowman S, Kaliner M (1984) Induction of human cutaneous mast cell degranulation by opiates and endogenous opioid peptides: evidence for opiate and nonopiate receptor participation. J Allergy Clin Immunol 73:775–781

Clement-Jones V, Lowry PJ, Rees JH, Besser GM (1980) Development of a specific extracted radioimmunoassay for methionine enkephalin in human plasma and cerebrospinal fluid. J Endocrinol 86:231–243

Duvaux-Meiret O, Stefano GB, Smith EM, Dissous C, Capron A (1992). Immunosuppression in the definitive and intermediate hosts of the human parasite Schistosoma mansoni by release of immunoactive neuropeptides. Proc Natl Acad Sci USA 89:778–781

Falke NE, Fischer EG (1986) Opiate receptor mediated internalization of ^{125}I-β-endorphin in human polymorphonuclear leucocytes. Cell Biol Int Rep 10:429–437

Finn JP, Steele LM, Barney PE, Eckroat LR (1991) Opioid involvement in the stimulation of conformational changes of immunocytes from the freshwater bivalve mollusc Proptera alata as revealed by light and scanning electron microscopy. Prog Neuroendocrine Immunol 4:180–186

Fischer EG, Falke NE (1984) β-Endorphin modulates immune functions—A review. Psychother Psychosom 42:195–204

Fischer EG, Falke NE (1986) The influence of endogenous opioid peptides on venous granulocytes. In: Plotnikoff NP, Faith RE, Murgo AJ, Good R (eds) Enkephalins and endorphins, stress and the immune system. Plenum, New York, pp 263–270

Heagy W, Laurance M, Cohen E, Finberg R (1990) Neurohormones regulate T-cell function. J Exp Med 171(5):1625–1633

Hughes TK Jr, Smith EM, Chin R, Cadet P, Sinisterra J, Leung MK, Shipp MA, Scharrer B, Stefano GB (1990) Interaction of immunoactive monokines (IL-1 and TNF) in the bivalve mollusc Mytilus edulis Proc Natl Acad Sci USA 87:4426–4429

Kimura T, Ota K, Matsui K, Iitake K, Shoji M, Inoue M, Yoshinaga K, Share L (1985) The presence of methionine-enkephalin in plasma and urine in normal human subjects and various patients. Endocrinol Jpn 32:514–517

Kornfeld H, Cruikshank WPS, Berman J, Center D (1985) Lymphocyte activation by HIV-1 envelope glycoprotein. Nature 335:445–448

Leung MK, Stefano GB (1987) Comparative neurobiology of opioids in invertebrates with special attention to senescent alterations. Prog Neurobiol 28:131–159

Lolait SJ, Lim ATW, Toh BH, Fimder JW (1984) Immunoreactive β-endorphin in a subpopulation of mouse spleen macrophages. J Clin Invest 73:277–280

Lolait SJ, Clements JA, Markwick AJ, Cheng C, Mc Nally M, Smith AI, Funder JW (1986) Proopiomelanocortin messenger ribonucleic acid and posttranslational processing of β-endorphin in spleen macrophages. J Clin Invest 77:1776–1781

Ottaviani E, Petraglia F, Montagnani G, Cossarizza A, Monti D (1990) Presence of ACTH and β-endorphin immunoreactive molecules in the freshwater snail Planorbarius corneus (L.) (Gastropoda, Pulmonata) and their possible role in phagocytosis. Regul Pept 27:1–9

Renwrantz L (1990) Internal defense system of Mytilus edulis. In: Stefano GB (ed) Neurobiology of *Mytilus edulis*. Manchester University Press, Manchester, pp 256–275

Ruff MR, Pert CB (1986) Neuropeptides are chemoattractants for human monocytes and tumor cells: A basis for mind–body communication. In: Plotnikoff NP, Faith RE, Murgo AJ, Good R (eds) Enkephalins and endorphins, stress and the immune system. Plenum Press, New York, pp 387–398

Saland LC, Van Epps DE, Ortiz E, Samora A (1983) Acute injections of opiate peptides into the rat cerebral ventricle; a macrophage-like cellular response. Brain Res Bull 10:523–528

Scharrer B (1972) Cytophysiological features of hemocytes in cockroaches. Z Zellforschung 129: 301–319

Schön JC, Torre-Bueno J, Stefano GB (1991) Microscopic computer-assisted analysis of conformational state: reference to neuroimmunology. Adv Neuroimmunol 1:252–259

Simpkins CO, Dickey CA, Fink MP (1984) Human neutrophil migration is enhanced by β-endorphin. Life Sci 34:2251–2255

Shipp MA, Stefano GB, D'Adamio L, Switzer SN, Howard FD, Sinisterra J, Scharrer B, Reinherz E (1990) CD10/neutral endopeptidase 24·11 ("enkephalinase") downregulates enkephalin-mediated inflammatory responses in invertebrate and mammalian organisms. Nature 347:394–396

Shipp MA, Stefano GB, Switzer SN, Griffin JD, Reinherz EL (1991) CD10 (CALLA)/neutral endopeptidase 24·11 modulates inflammatory peptide-induced changes in neutrophil morphology, migration, and adhesion proteins and is itself regulated by neutrophil activation. Blood 78:1834–1841

Smith EM, Blalock JE (1981) Human lymphocyte production of corticotropin and endorphin-like substances: association with leukocyte interferon. Proc Natl Acad Sci USA 78:7530–7535

Smith EM, Hughes TK, Hashemi F, Stefano GB (1992) Immunosuppressive effects of ACTH and MSH and their possible significane in human immunodeficiency virus infection. Proc Natl Acad Sci USA 89:782–786

Stefano GB (1986) Conformational matching: a determining force in maintaining signal molecules. In: Stefano GB (ed) Comp. opioid and related neuropeptide mechanisms, vol 2. CRC Press, Boca Raton, pp 271–277

Stefano GB (1988) The evolvement of signal systems: conformational matching a determining force stabilizing families of signal molecules. Comp Biochem Physiol 90C:287–294

Stefano GB (1989) Role of opioid neuropeptides in immunoregulation. Prog Neurobiol 33:149–159

Stefano GB (1991) Conformational matching a stabilizing signal system factor during evolution: additional evidence in comparative neuroimmunology. Adv Neuroimmunol 1:71–82

Stefano GB, Leung MK, Zhao X, Scharrer B (1989a) Evidence for the involvement of opioid neuropeptides in the adherence and migration of immunocompetent invertebrate hemocytes. Proc Natl Acad Sci USA 86:626–630

Stefano GB, Cadet P, Scharrer B (1989b) Stimulatory effects of opioid neuropeptides on locomotory activity and conformational changes in invertebrate and human immunocytes: evidence for a subtype of delta receptor. Proc Natl Acad Sci USA 86:6307–6311

Stefano GB, Shipp MA, Scharrer B (1991a) A possible immunoregulatory function for Met-enkephalin-Arg^6-Phe^7 involving human and invertebrate granulocytes, 31:97–103

Stefano GB, Smith DM, Smith EM, Hughes TK (1991b) MSH can deactivate both TNF stimulated and spontaneously active immunocytes. In: Molluscan neurobiology. Kits KS, Boer HH, Joosse J (eds) North Holland, Amsterdam, pp 206–209

Taché Y, Morley JE, Brown MR (eds) (1989) Neuropeptides and stress. Springer, Berlin, Heidelberg, New York

Van Epps DE, Mason MM (1990) Modulation of leukocyte migration by α melanocyte stimulating hormone. In: Florey E, Stefano GB (eds) Comparative neuropeptide pharmacology. Manchester University Press, Manchester, pp 335–345

Van Epps DE, Saland LC (1984) β-Endorphin and Met-enkephalin stimulate peripheral blood mononuclear cell chemotaxis. J Immunol 132:3046–3053

Van Epps DE, Durant DA, Potter JW (1983) Migration of human helper/inducer T cells in response to supernatants from con-A-stimulated suppressor/cytotoxic T cells. J Immunol 131:697–703

Van Ree JM, Bohus B, Csontos KM, Gispen WH, Greven HM, Nijkamp FP, Opmeer FA, De Rotte AA, Van Wimersma Greidanus TB, Witter A, De Wied D (1981) Behavioral profile of γ-MSH: relationship with ACTH and β-endorphin. Life Sci 28:2875–2888

Zurawski G, Benedik M, Kamb BJ, Abrams JS, Zurawski SM, Lee FD (1986) Activation of mouse T-helper cells induces abundant preproenkephalin mRNA synthesis. Science 232:772–775

Role of Neuropeptides in the Bidirectional Communication Between the Immune and Neuroendocrine Systems

D. A. Weigent and J. E. Blalock

Introduction

Vertebrates respond to infection and inflammation with a complex series of intercellular communication signals involving the immune, nervous, and endocrine systems. Recent investigations have shown that the immune system is subject to neural and endocrine control, and that it exerts in turn a reciprocal effect on the nervous system. In addition, the immune system is capable of producing neuropeptides, and the nervous system is able to secrete cytokines. This chapter summarizes the evidence for the production and function of neuropeptides in this regulatory relationship. The neuropeptides discussed here include corticotropin (ACTH), β-endorphin, vasoactive intestinal peptide (VIP), somatostatin (SOM), and substance P. Overall, a rapidly expanding body of evidence indicates that neuropeptides and cytokines are the common signal molecules that mediate bidirectional communication between the immune and neuroendocrine systems.

Production of Neuropeptides by Cells of the Immune System

Table 1 summarizes the production of neuropeptides by cells of the immune system. The demonstration of neuropeptide-mediated alterations of immune response depends on whether the appropriate ligand can be identified at the appropriate site. Findings from our laboratory and others have provided evidence for direct neural communication via neuropeptides with cells of the immune system as well as the ability of lymphocytes to produce neuropeptides. Thus, immunohistochemical methods have revealed the presence of numerous neuropeptides in primary and secondary lymphoid organs, including substance P, VIP, neuropeptide Y, enkephalin, endorphin, cholecystokinin, vasopressin, calcium gene-related peptide, and SOM (Bellinger et al. 1990). Similarly to

University of Alabama at Birmingham, Department of Physiology and Biophysics, UAB Station, Birmingham, AL 35294–0001, USA

Scharrer et al. (Eds.)
Neuropeptides and Immunoregulation

Table 1. Neuropeptides produced by cells of the immune system

Hormone	Inducer	Cell type	Reference
ACTH and endorphins	Newcastle disease virus	T, B, mac	Blalock and Smith (1980)
			Smith and Blalock (1981)
	LPS	B	Harbour-McMenamin et al. (1985)
	CRF	—	Smith et al. (1986)
VIP		PMNs	Lygren et al. (1984)
		Mast cells	Goetzl et al. (1990a)
Substance P		Eosinophils	Weinstock and Blum (1989)
Somatostatin		PMNs	Lygren et al. (1984)
			Fuller and Verity (1989)
GHRH	Constitutive	—	Weigent and Blalock (1990)
LHRH	Constitutive	—	Marchetti et al. (1990)

noradrenergic sympathetic innervation of lymphoid organs, peptidergic nerve fibers distribute with the vasculature into parenchymal fields of lymphocytes. It is possible that the target T-cells become either activated or suppressed by certain neuropeptides.

Cells of the immune system may become exposed to neurohormones as a result of their secretion from the hypothalamic-pituitary axis or from cells of the immune system. It has been shown that T-lymphocytes produce ACTH, β-endorphin, corticotropin-releasing hormone (CRH), and growth hormone-releasing hormone (GHRH) while eosinophils produce VIP and substance P. Taken together, the in vitro studies suggest that VIP-related peptides from mast T-cells and basophils, SOM-like peptides from monocytes and mast T-cells, and ACTH from lymphocytes, macrophages, and mast T-cells can be structurally different from previously defined neuropeptides (Harbour-McMenamin et al. 1985; Harbour et al. 1987; Goetzl et al. 1988, 1990a). The isolation of distinctive fragments of VIP from lymphocytes supports the idea of post-translational peptidolysis in the generation of this diversity (Harbour-McMenamin et al. 1985; Harbour et al. 1987; Goetzl et al. 1991). The substance P generated in granulomas of murine schistosomiasis is attributable to eosinophils, as shown by the localization of substance P immunoreactivity and mRNA (Weinstock and Blum 1990).

The evidence for the production of neuroendocrine hormones by cells of the immune system has been obtained by showing the presence of specific mRNA molecules and peptide products with properties similar to those of neuronal origin. These include ACTH and/or endorphins (Blalock and Smith 1980; Harbour-McMenamin et al. 1985; Westley et al. 1986; Oates et al. 1988; Buzzetti et al. 1989; Ferreira et al. 1990), thyroid-stimulating hormone (TSH; Smith et al. 1983; Harbour et al. 1987), prolactin (Hiestand et al. 1986), growth hormone (GH; Weigent et al. 1988), and more recently the releasing hormones CRH (Hargreaves et al. 1989; Stephanou et al. 1990) and GHRH (Weigent and Blalock 1990); The bioactivity, molecular weight, and antigenicity of the leukocyte-derived hormones indicate identity with their neural counterparts. The production of several of these hormones by lymphocytes is discussed in greater detail below.

ACTH was the first de novo synthesized hormone shown to be produced by the immune system. This occurred when it was observed that both human and mouse leukocytes expressed an ACTH-like peptide following virus infection or in the presence of transformed cells or bacterial lipopolysaccaride (Harbour-McMenamin et al. 1985). An important finding (Smith and Blalock 1981) was that virus infection of hypophysectomized animals stimulated the production of an ACTH-like substance which could be blocked by dexamethasone (Smith et al. 1982). Subsequently, other workers have reported the presence of ACTH-like activity in the immune system (Healy et al. 1983; Lolait et al. 1984, 1986; Westley et al. 1986; Oates et al. 1988). Northern blot analysis of mouse and rat spleen poly(A) mRNA clearly showed that pro-opiomelanocortin (POMC) RNA is generated within the spleen (Lolait et al. 1986). Expression of the POMC gene has been reported in normal human lymphocytes and lymphocyte cell lines infected with lymphotropic viruses (Oates et al. 1988). More recent data conclusively demonstrate that T-lymphocytes produce authentic ACTH and harbor its RNA. The lymphocyte mRNA has been reverse transcribed, cloned, sequenced, and shown to be identical with that of mouse pituitary ACTH precursor (Smith et al. 1990).

An interesting feature concerning lymphocyte POMC mRNA is the absence of exons 1 and 2 from the three exons which make up the POMC gene. Mouse splenic mononuclear leukocytes have been found to transcribe at least two truncated transcripts of exon 3 (Galin et al. 1991). The significance of the absence of exons 1 and 2 of the POMC gene in lymphocytes and the presence of multiple forms of exon 3 transcripts is unknown although it is tempting to speculate that the protein products may play an important role during normal and/or inflammatory processes.

With regard to processing of the precursor, the data indicate the existence of an alternate processing pathway for the POMC molecule. Thus, CRH was shown to stimulate production of ACTH (1–39) and β-endorphin by lymphocytes while lipopolysaccharide (LPS) was shown to induce de novo synthesis of a smaller (2.9 kDa) ACTH (1–25) molecule plus α- and γ-endorphin (Harbour-McMenamin et al. 1985). A novel enzyme active at pH 5 can be isloated from LPS-treated B-lymphocyte lysates that cleave ACTH (1–39) (4·5 kDa) to a smaller fragment (2·9 kDa; Harbour et al. 1987). The results indicate a unique processing pathway within the immune system which may play an important role in the pathophysiology of endotoxic shock (Harbour-McMenamin et al. 1985). The precise molecular identity of the ACTH-like peptide from lymphocytes with pituitary ACTH has also been established at the amino acid level. The results show that the amino acid sequence is identical with that of ACTH (1–25) (Smith et al. 1990).

The extrahypothalamic production of hypothalamic releasing hormones has been well documented. It has been reported that the human placenta contains several kinds of hypothalamic releasing hormones such as corticotropin-releasing factor (CRF; Shibasaki et al. 1982; Sasaki et al. 1987), thyrotropin-releasing hormone (TRH; Gibbons et al. 1975) and luteining hormone-releasing hormone (LHRH; Gibbons et al. 1975; Khodr and Siler-Khodr 1980). The presence of immunoreactive and biologically active GHRH in rat placenta has also been described (Sasaki et al. 1989). The source of GHRH in plasma is uncertain, and irGHRH is present in extrahypothalamic areas of the brain, in lung, liver, pancreas, and in the gastrointestinal tract (Shibasaki et al. 1984). The first report showing expression of a hypothalamic releasing hormone by cells of the immune system was for GHRH (Weigent and, Blalock 1990). Thus by RNA slot-blot analysis, maximum basal levels of specific GHRH mRNA in the cytoplasm of rat leukocytes were detected after an 8-h in vitro incubation. Northern gel analysis demonstrated the specific GHRH RNA which contained approximately 0·8 kb. Further studies with antibody-affinity chromatography followed by size separation on high-pressure liquid chromatography columns showed two peaks of ir material, a large molecular weight species, and a smaller molecular weight species at approximately 5 kDa. The smaller molecular weight irGHRH appeared to be synthesized de novo since it could be radiolabeled with tritiated amino acids. Most importantly, the lower molecular weight leukocyte-derived GHRH could block the binding of ^{125}I-labeled hGHRH to pituitary cells and stimulate an increase in the level of GH RNA in the pituitary.

Also very recently it has been suggested that LHRH is expressed by immune cells (Marchetti et al. 1990). Poly (A+) mRNA from murine thymocytes and splenocytes was used as a template for selective cDNA synthesis and polymerase chain reaction (PCR). Amplification primers were designed to yield a 330-bp cDNA product. PCR products from thymocyte and splenocyte mRNA preparations with an LHRH-specific ^{32}P-labeled oligodeoxynucleotide probe showed that the coding sequence for LHRH was present. Finally, the release of a substance from inflamed tissue similar to CRF has been described (Hargreaves et al. 1989). Additional studies by in situ hybridization have demonstrated CRF mRNA in T- and B-lymphocytes and in neutrophils. Northern blot analysis has revealed the presence of CRF mRNA species of 1·7 kb from lymphocytes, and a peptide that reacts with anti-CRF antiserum was identified by radioimmunoassay (Stephanou et al. 1990). Taken together, these findings demonstrate a potential regulatory loop utilizing hypothalamic releasing hormones between the immune and neuroendocrine tissues.

Lymphocyte Receptors for Neuropeptides

An important finding supporting the idea that neuropeptides influence the immune system comes from data showing functional receptors for neuropeptides on cells of the immune system. Thus, receptors for VIP have been reported on human peripheral blood mononuclear cells (Guerrero et al. 1981) and murine

T- and B-lymphocytes (Ottaway and Greenberg 1984). The affinity of binding of ^{125}I-labeled VIP1–10 by mammalian liver, cerebral cortex, and pituitary is one order of magnitude higher than that seen in lymphocytes (Goetzl et al. 1990b). Although the affinity and specificity of the combining sites of VIP receptors on neurons and lymphoid cells differ, the major protein component is similar. The electrophoretic characterization after radioactive affinity labeling and chromatographic analysis of solubilized binding sites have revealed a monomeric protein of approximately 50 KDa in Mot 4B-lymphocytes and in mammalian lung, cerebral cortex, and liver cells (Goetzl et al. 1990a; Wenger and O'Dorisio 1990).

Receptors for substance P have been described on human (Payan et al. 1984a) and murine (Stanisz et al. 1987b) lymphocytes and rat peritoneal mast cells (Piotrowski et al. 1987). The end of the substance P molecule at the carboxy-terminal is important in ligand binding to lymphocytes (Payan et al. 1983), while the amino-terminal end is necessary for release of mediators in inflammation (Goetzl et al. 1985). Receptors for SOM have been reported on human monocytes and lymphocytes (Bhathena et al. 1981), murine T- and B-lymphocytes (Stanisz et al. 1987b), and basophils (Goetzl and Payan 1984).

Cells of the immune system also possess receptors for ACTH, CRF, and opiate/opioid (Weigent and Blalock 1987). For example, binding studies have shown that mouse spleen cell populations have two binding affinities for ACTH, one a high-affinity (kDa 0.1 n*M*) and the other a low-affinity (kDa 4·8 n*M*) receptor (Johnson et al. 1982). These seem to correspond in molecular weight to high (k_d 0.25 n*M*) and low affinity (k_d 10 n*M*) receptors on rat adrenal cells (McIlhinney and Schulster 1975). A comparison of the average number of binding sites per cell shows approximately 3000 high- and 50 000 low-affinity sites on splenocytes compared to 3000 high- and 30 000 low-affinity sites on adrenal cells. Using a new technology for the development of antiserum specific for the ACTH receptor, we showed that the receptor for ACTH has a total molecular weight of 225 kDa and is composed of four polypeptide chains of 83, 64, 52, and 22 kDa, respectively. The purified receptor possesses binding affinities of $3.4 \times 10^{10} M^{-1}$ and $1.0 \times 10^{9} M^{-1}$ as determined by Scatchard analysis, The ACTH-binding site was located on the 83 kDa polypeptide chain (Bost and Blalock 1985). Opioid receptors have also been demonstrated on cells of the immune system (Weigent and Blalock 1987; see also Stefano, this volume).

CRF receptors were first identified on pituitary corticotropic cells conveying stimuli for the synthesis of POMC and subsequent secretion of ACTH (Rivier and Plotsky 1986). In addition to various immunostimulants (e.g., virus infection, LPS), synthetic CRF at nanomolar concentrations was able to stimulate peripheral blood mononuclear leukocytes to synthesize ACTH and β-endorphin (Woloski et al. 1985). Over 50% of the cells could be induced to express POMC-derived peptides with 10 n*M* vasopressin augmenting this response. The suppression of CRF-receptor-induced ACTH expression by dexamethasone suggests that regulation of the respective gene might also be similar in leukocytes and pituitary cells. It is not presently known which subtypes of cells express CRF receptors. Circulating lymphocytes passing through the hypothalamic-hypophysial portal vessels may be exposed to releasing hormones such as CRF (Antoni 1986). It may be here or at extrahypothalamic sites of CRF production (Yasuda et al. 1982) that these receptors bind ligand. The importance of CRF receptors on leukocytes may be a mechanism by which local levels of ACTH of other POMC-derived peptides are elevated and thereby able to function within lymphoid organs.

Effect of Neuropeptides on Immune Cells

Most interactions between the neuroendocrine and immune systems have been attributed to the effects of glucocorticoid hormones via induction by ACTH. More recently, however , it has become clear that neuropeptides can directly modulate the immune response. A summary of a few examples is shown in Table 2 and discussed below for ACTH, endorphins, substance P, SOM, and VIP.

ACTH has been found to regulate the functions of the major types of cells within the immune system. In an in vitro plaque-forming cell assay, ACTH (1–39) suppressed the response to both a T-cell-dependent antigen (sheep red blood cells) and a T-lymphocyte-independent antigen (dinitrophenol-Ficoll; Johnson et al. 1982). For maximal inhibition of antibody synthesis it was necessary for

Table 2. Immunoregulatory effects of neuropeptides

Hormone	Immunologic Function	Reference
ACTH	Suppresses Ig and IFN-γ synthesis	Johnson et al. (1982)
	Augments B-cell proliferation	Alverez-Mon et al. (1985)
	Suppresses macrophage activation	Koff and Dunegan (1985)
β-Endorphin	Enhances Ig and IFN-γ synthesis	Brown and Van Epps (1986); Heijnen et al. (1986)
	Enhances NK cell activity	Froelich and Bankhurst (1984)
	Chemotactic for monocytes	Ruff et al. (1985)
	Enhances CTL	Carr and Klimpel (1986)
VIP	Alters antibody production	Stanisz et al. (1986)
	Inhibits mitogen-induced proliferation	Ottaway and Greenburg (1985)
	Influences lymphocyte migration	Ottaway (1984)
Substance P	Stimulates mitogen-induced proliferation	Stanisz et al. (1986)
	Stimulates histamine release	Goetzl et al. (1985)
Somatostatin	Inhibits mitogen-induced proliferation	Stanisz et al. (1987a)
	Stimulates chemotaxis	Ruff et al. (1985)
	Stimulates neutrophil phagocytosis	Bar Shavit et al. (1980)
GHRH	Proliferation	Bozzola et al. (1987)
	Stimulates NK	Pawlikoski et al. (1988)
	Stimulates chemotaxis	Zalazowski et al. (1989)

ACTH (1–39) to be present at the time of antigen addition, and thiol-reducing agents blocked the ACTH-mediated effect. The mechanism by which ACTH inhibits the antibody response may be similar to that of interferon (IFN) since these characteristics are associated with the inhibition of antibody synthesis by IFN-α and -β (Johnson et al. 1982). In contrast to the inhibitory effects of ACTH on antibody production in the murine spleen cell system, ACTH enhances the growth and differentiation of enriched cultures of human tonsillar B-cells (Alvarez-Mon et al. 1985). Furthermore, ACTH enhances interleukin (IL)-2 and B-cell differentiation factor-induced IgM and IgG secretion by activated B-cells at concentrations similar to those for enhancement of proliferation. Thus, it appears that ACTH may either enhance or inhibit B-cell function, probably depending on factors such as ACTH concentration, source of B-cells, presence of other factors such as lymphokines, and presence of accessory T-cells. T-cell and macrophage functions are also modulated by ACTH. For instance, this hormone suppressed in vitro IFN-γ production (Johnson et al. 1984) by T-lymphocytes. In addition to blocking the T-cell production of IFN-γ, ACTH completely blocked the ability of preformed IFN-γ to activate macrophages to a tumoricidal state (Koff and Dunnegan 1985). Thus, ACTH is able to modulate the function of each of the principal cell types within the immune system.

The production of ACTH by lymphocytes is associated with that of production of endorphin-like substances. Opioid peptides have been shown to influence the functions of cells within the immune system following opioid peptide administration either in vivo or in vitro. Briefly, opioid peptides suppress antibody production (Johnson et al. 1982; Heijnen et al. 1986; Hadjupetrou-Kourounakis et al. 1989), enhance leukocyte chemotaxis (Van Epps and Saland 1984), augment macrophage antibody-dependent cytotoxicity (Foris et al. 1984), enhance IFN-γ production by human peripheral blood mononuclear cells (Brown and Van Epps 1986), enhance mitogen-induced lymphocyte proliferation (Gilman et al. 1982), increase IL-1 induced IL-2 production (Bessler et al. 1990), augment the generation of cytotoxic T-lymphocytes (Carr and Klimpel 1986), and enhance natural killer cell (NK) activity (Mathews et al. 1983; Oleson and Johnson 1988).

Hypothalamic releasing hormones have been shown to modulate the immune system. CRH induces the production of irACTH and endorphin by lymphocytes (Smith et al. 1986). This early observation was recently supported by the finding that subcutaneous administration of CRH (50 μg/kg) elicited β-endorphin production by lymphocytes taken from the spleen and mesenteric lymph nodes (Kavelaars et al. 1990b). Moreover, the production of the POMC-derived peptides elicited by CRH is inhibited by the negative feedback inhibitor glucocorticoid (Kavelaars et al. 1990a) which reportedly acts by abrogating IL-1 production which in turn is responsible for β-endorphin production (Kavelaars et al. 1989). CRH has also been shown to increase IL-2 receptor expression on T-lymphocytes and to stimulate lymphocyte proliferation in the presence or absence of mitogens (Singh 1989). Moreover, CRH has been shown to enhance NK cytolytic activity of splenocytes in a naloxone-reversible manner. This indicates that CRH acts indirectly on NK cells through its ability to induce β-endorphin production (Carr et al. 1990). Collectively, CRH acts in the immune system through an intricate network encompassing selective target T-cells and eliciting the release of specific cytokines.

Other hypothalamic releasing hormones which are active in the immune system include GHRH, LHRH, and TRH. GHRH has been shown to increase GH mRNA in leukocytes and to cause a two-fold increase in thymidine and uridine incorporation of unstimulated lymphocytes (Guarcello, unpublished). GHRH also stimulates lymphocyte proliferation (Bozzola et al. 1987), inhibits NK activity (Pawlikowski et al. 1988), and inhibits the chemotactic response (Zelazowski et al. 1989). LHRH administered in vivo to hypophysectomized animals reportedly stimulates thymic hypertrophy and thymocyte proliferation but not in untreated animals (Marchetti et al. 1989). In addition, LHRH has been shown to reverse thymic atrophy and thymocyte proliferation in aged animals (Marchetti et al. 1989). Finally, TRH enhances antibody production indirectly by stimulating TSH production, which has previously been shown to augment antibody production (Kruger et al. 1989). Thus, hypothalamic releasing hormones are produced by immune cells and influence immunological functions.

Neuropeptides such as VIP, substance P, and SOM are potent mediators of many of the activities of cells of the immune system. VIP can alter antibody production (Stanisz et al. 1986). VIP can inhibit mitogen-induced proliferation of lymphocytes from murine Peyer's patches and spleen (Ottaway and Greenberg 1984) and inhibit NK activity (Rola-Pleszczynski et al. 1985). VIP also influences the migration of T-lymphocytes into gut-associated lymphoid tissue (Ottaway 1984) and mesenteric lymph nodes (Moore 1984). Preincubation of rat T-lymphocytes from Peyer's patches with VIP, in concentrations that downregulate VIP receptors on T-lymphocytes prevents homing of desensitized T-lymphocytes to Peyer's patches following adoptive transfer of these cells into a syngeneic host (Ottaway 1984). VIP also appears to be involved in vasodilatation of vascular beds during local inflammatory responses (Payan et al. 1984c).

Substance P stimulates mitogen-induced proliferation of lymphocytes (Stanisz et al. 1986), stimulates lymphocyte proliferation, plays a major role in local inflammation via dilation of vascular beds (Lundbert et al. 1983), and stimulates mast cells and basophils to release histamine and other mediators such a leukotrienes (Goetzl et al. 1985).

In addition, SOM can influence several immune functions in vitro, including concentration-dependent modulation of spontaneous proliferation of murine splenocytes (Pawlikowski et al. 1985), inhibition of mitogen-stimulated proliferation of murine splenocytes (Stanisz et al. 1987a), human T-lymphocytes, and Molt-4b human lymphoblast cell line (Payan et al. 1984b), and reduction in colony-stimulating activity of murine splenocytes (Theoharides and Douglas 1981). SOM is also a major mediator of immediate hypersensitivity through its stimulation of leukocyte and monocyte chemotaxis (Ruff et al. 1985), neutrophil phagocytosis (Bar-Shavit et al. 1980), and release of histamine and leukotrienes by basophils and mast T-cells (Shanahan et al. 1985).

Neuropeptides alter the effects of some cytokines (Goetzl 1990b). For example, nanomolar concentrations of substance P, substance K, and neurokinins A and B evoke the generation of IL-1, TNF-α, and IL-6 by mononuclear phagocytes. Also, α-MSH selectively blocks the stimulation of thymocytes by IL-1 in vitro and the inflammatory effects of IL-1 and TNF in mice. Arginine vasopressin replaces helper T-cells in the generation of IFN-γ by mouse spleen lymphocytes (Johnson and Torres 1985). T-cells produce proteins that influence the growth and differentiation of various neural cells. In a few instances, the purified factors appear to be directed to astrocytes and others to oligodendrocytes (Merrill et al. 1984). Thus, neuropeptides in these complex tissue reactions may indirectly influence the growth of neural cells via substances secreted by leukocytes.

Summary

Neuropeptides, produced by cells of the immune system as well as neuronal and additional cell types, participate in the regulation of important immune functions (see Tables 1, 2). The effects of neuropeptide signals, dispatched by either source and received by immune cells via neuropeptide receptors, include: (a) enhancement and suppression of antibody production; (b) enhancement and suppression of lymphocyte cytotoxicity and proliferation; (c) modulation of lymphokine production and mediation of lymphokine function; (d) initiation of hypersensitivity events and possibly some immune complex diseases; (e) modulation of macrophage and neutrophil functions; and (f) enhancement of primary lymphoid organ function such as thymic regeneration. The production and secretion of these hormones by leukocytes is similar in some respects and different in others from that observed in neuroendocrine cells.

Conversely, neuropeptides released from immune cells transmit information to the nervous system. It is our opinion that the transmission of information to the nervous system represents a sensory function of the immune system wherein leukocytes recognize stimuli that are not recognized by the central and peripheral nervous systems (Blalock 1984; Fig. 1). These stimuli have been termed noncognitive and include those brought about by bacteria, tumors, viruses, and antigens. The recognition of such noncognitive stimuli by immunocytes is then converted into information conveyed to the nervous system by peptide hormones, lymphokines, and monokines resulting in physiological changes. A better understanding of the interactions between the nervous and immune systems will have both theoretical and practical implications in our appreciation of the immune response to disease.

We expect that in the immediate future the structural relationship of lymphocyte-derived neuropeptides with their neural counterparts will be firmly established. In addition, we expect that the mechanisms regulating the synthesis and secretion of neuropeptides by immune cells will become known. Ultimately,

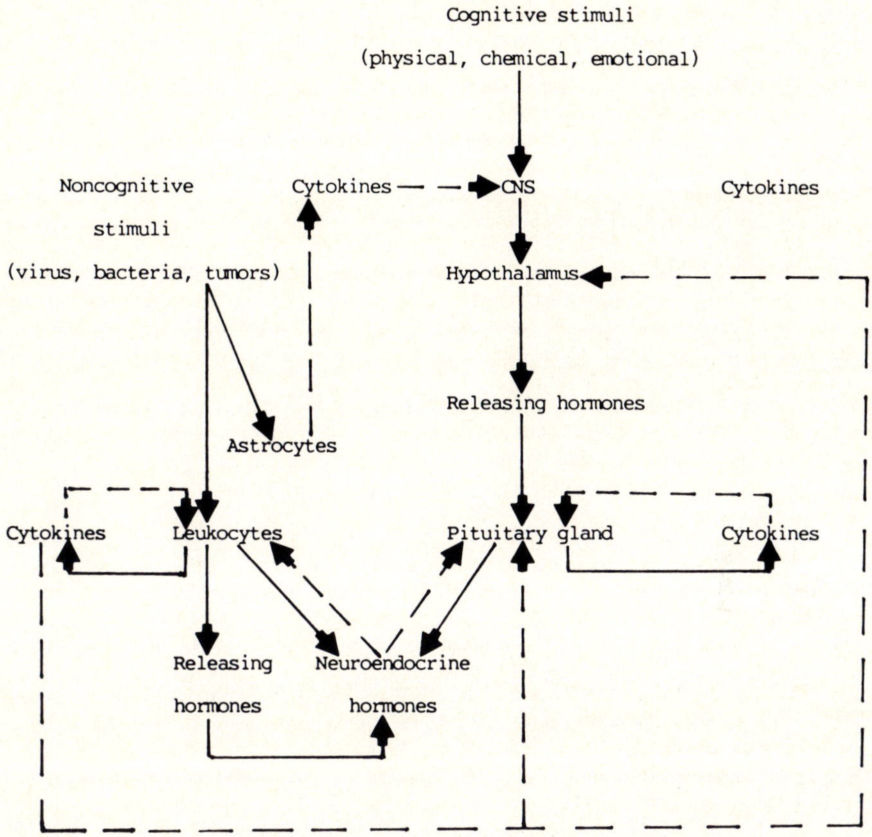

Fig. 1 Mediation of signals between the immune system and the neuroendocrine system by neuropeptides and cytokines

such information may be useful in addressing the role(s) of these molecules in immunological, neurological, and behavioral diseases.

Acknowledgements. This work was supported, in part, by NIH grants RO1 DK38024 and RO1 NS24636 and Council for Tobacco Research-USA grant 2222. The authors are indebted to former and present colleagues for their excellent contributions to these studies. We also thank Diane Weigent for typing this manuscript as well as excellent editorial assistance.

References

Alvarez-Mon A, Kehrl JH, Fauci AS (1985) A potential role for adrenocorticotropin in regulating human B-lymphocyte functions. J Immunol 135:3823–3826

Antoni FA (1986) Hypothalamic control of ACTH secretion. Endocr Rec 2:351–378

Bar-Shavit Z, Goldman R, Stabinsky Y, Gottleib F, Fridkin M, Teichberg V, Blumberg S (1980) Enhancement of phagocytosis— a newly found activity of substance P residing in its N- terminal tetrapeptide sequence. Biochem Biophys Res Commun 94:1445–1451

Bellinger DL, Lorton D, Romano TD, Olschowka JA, Felten SY, Felten DL (1990) Neuropeptide innervation of lymphoid organs. Ann NY Acad Sci 594:17–33

Bessler H, Sztein MB, Serrate SA (1990) β-Endorphin modulation of IL-1 induced IL-2 production. Immunopharmacology 19:5–14

Bhathena SJ, Louie J, Schechter GP, Redman RS, Wahl L, Recant L (1981) Identification of human mononuclear leukocytes bearing receptors for somatostatin and glucagon. Diabetes 30: 127–131

Blalock JE (1984) The immune system as a sensory organ. J Immunol 132:1067–1070

Blalock JE, Smith EM (1980) Human leukocyte interferon: structural and biological relatedness to adrenocorticotropic hormone and endorphins. Proc Natl Acad Sci USA 77:5972–5974

Bost KL, Blalock JE (1985) Molecular characterization of a corticotropin (ACTH) receptor. Mol Cell Endocrinol 44:1–9

Bozzola M, Moretta A, Maccario R, Bohen M, Burgio GR (1987) Modulating effect of growth hormone (GH) on in vitro lymphoproliferation. 1st European congress on endocrinology, Copenhagen, abstract no 148

Brown SL, Van Epps D (1986) Opioid peptides modulate production of interferon-γ by human mononuclear cells. Cell Immunol 103:19–26

Buzzetti R, McLoughlin L, Lavender PM, Clark AJL, Rees LH (1989) Expression of proopiomelanocortin gene and quantification of adrenocorticotropic hormone-like immuno-reactivity in human normal peripheral mononuclear cells and lymphoid and myeloid malignancies. J Clin Invest 83:733–737

Carr DJJ, Klimpel GR (1986) Enhancement of the generation of cytotoxic T-cells by endogenous opiates. J Neuroimmunol 12:75–87

Carr DJJ, DeCosta BR, Jacobson AE, Rice KC, Blalock JE (1990) Corticotropin-releasing hormone augments natural killer cell activity through a naloxone-sensitive pathway. J Neuroimmunol 28:53–61

Ferreira JA, Carstens ME, Taljaard JJF (1990) Quantitative determination of lymphocyte ACTH-1–39. Neuropeptides 15:11–15

Foris G, Medgyesi GA, Gyimesi E, Hauck M (1984) Met-enkephalin induced alterations of macrophage functions. Mol Immunol 21:747–750

Froelich OJ, Bankhurst AD (1984) The effect of beta-endorphin on natural cytotoxicity and antibody-dependent cellular cytotoxicity. Life Sci 35:261–265

Fuller PJ, Verity K (1989) Somatostatin gene expression in the thymus gland. J Immunol 143: 1015–1017

Galin FS, LeBoeuf RD, Blalock JE (1991) Corticotropin releasing factor unregulates expression of two truncated pro-opiomelanocortin transcripts in lymphocytes. J Neuroimmunol 31: 51–58

Gibbons JM, Mitnick M, Chieffo V (1975) In vitro biosynthesis of TSH and LH-releasing factors by the human placenta. Am J Obstet Gynecol 121:127–131

Gilman SC, Schwartz JM, Milner RJ, Bloom FE, Feldman JD (1982) β-Endorphin enhances lymphocyte proliferative responses. Proc Natl Acad Sci USA 79:4226–4230

Goetzl EJ, Payan DG (1984) Inhibition by somatostatin of the release of mediators from human basophils and rat leukemic basophils. J Immunol 133:3255–3259

Goetzl EJ, Chernov T, Renold F, Payan DG (1985) Neuropeptide regulation of the expression of immediate hypersensitivity. J Immunol 135:802S–805S

Goetzl EJ, Sreedharan SP, Turck DW (1988) Structurally distinctive vasoactive intestinal peptides from rat basophilic leukemia cells. J Biol Chem 263:9083–9086

Goetzl EJ, Grotmol T, Van Dyke RW, Turck CW, Wershil B, Galli SJ, Sreedharan SP (1990a) Generation and recognition of vasoactive intestinal peptide by cells of the immune system. Ann NY Acad Sci 594:34–44

Goetzl EJ, Adelman DC, Sreedharan SP (1990b) Neuroimmunology. In: Dixon FJ, Austen KF, Hood L, Uhr UW (eds) Advances in immunology. Academic Press, New York

Goetzl EJ, Turck C, Sreedharan S (1991) Production and recognition of neuropeptides by cells of the immune system. In: Ader R, Cohen N, Felten DL (eds) Psychoneuroimmunology, 2nd edn. Academic, New York, pp 263–282

Guerrero JM, Prieto JC, Elorza FL, Ramirez R, Goberna R (1981) Interaction of vasoactive intestinal peptide with human blood mononuclear cells. Mol Cell Endocrinol 21:151–160

Hadjupetrou-Kourounakis L, Karagounis E, Rekka E, Kourounakis P (1989) Immunosuppression by a novel opioid agonist. Scand J Immunol 29:449–458

Harbour DV, Smith EM, Blalock JE (1987) A novel processing pathway for proopiomelanocortin in lymphocytes: endotoxin induction of a new prohormone-cleaving enzyme. J Neurosci Res 18:95–101

Harbour-McMenamin DV, Smith EM, Blalock JE (1985) Endotoxin induction of leukocyte-derived proopiomelanocortin related peptides. Infect Immun 48:813–819

Hargreaves KM, Costello AH, Joris JL (1987) Release from inflamed tissue of a substance with properties similar to corticotropin-releasing factor. Neuroendocrinology 49:476–482

Healy DL, Hodgen GD, Schulte HM, Chrousos GP, Loriaux DL, Hall NR, Goldstein AL (1983) The thymus adrenal connection: thymosin has corticotropin releasing activity in primates. Science 222:1353–1355

Heijnen CJ, Bevers C, Kavelaars A, Ballieux RE (1986) Effect of α-endorphin on the antigen-induced primary antibody response of human blood B-cells in vitro. J Immunol 136:213–216

Hiestand PC, Mekler P, Nordmann R, Grieder A, Permmongkol C (1986) Prolactin as a modulator of lymphocyte responsiveness provides a possible mechanism of action for cyclosporin. Proc Natl Acad Sci USA 83:2599–2603

Johnson HM, Torres BA (1985) Regulation of lymphokine production by arginine vasopressin and oxytocin: modulation of lymphocyte function by neurohypophyseal hormones. J Immunol 135:773s–775s

Johnson HM, Smith EM, Torres BA, Blalock JE (1982) Neuroendocrine hormone regulation of in vitro antibody production. Proc Natl Acad Sci USA 79:4171–4174

Johnson HM, Torres BA, Smith EM, Dion LD, Blalock JE (1984) Regulation of lymphokine (interferon-γ) production by corticotropin. J Immunol 132:246–250

Kavelaars A, Ballieux RE, Heijnen CJ (1989) The role of IL-1 in the corticotropin-releasing factor and arginine vasopressin-induced secretion of immunoreactive β-endorphin by human peripheral blood mononuclear cells. J Immunol 142:2338–2342

Kavelaars A, Ballieux RE, Heijnen CJ (1990a) β-Endorphin secretion by human peripheral blood mononuclear cells: regulation by glucocorticoids. Life Sci 46:1233–1240

Kavelaars A, Berkenbosch F, Croiset G, Ballieux RE, Heijnen CJ (1990b) Induction of β-endorphin secretion by lymphocytes after subcutaneous administration of corticotropin-releasing factor. Endocrinology 126:759–764

Khodr GS, Siler-Khodr TM (1980) Placental luteinizing hormone-releasing factor and its synthesis. Science 207:315–317

Koff WC, Dunegan MA (1985) Modulation of macrophage-mediated tumoricidal activity by neuropeptides and neurohormones. J Immunol 135:350–354

Kruger TE, Smith LR, Harbour DV, Blalock JE (1989) Thyrotropin: an endogenous regulator of the in vitro immune response. J Immunol 142:744–747

Lolait SJ, Lim ATW, Toh BH, Funder JW (1984) Immunoreactive β-endorphin in a subpopulation of mouse spleen macrophages. J Clin Invest 73:277–280

Liolait SJ, Clements JA, Markwick AJ, Cheng C, McNally M, Smith AI, Funder JW (1986) Proopiomelanocortin messenger ribonucleic acid and posttranslational processing of β-endorphin in spleen macrophages. J Clin Invest 77:1776–1779

Lundbert JM, Saria A, Brodin E, Rossell S, Folkars K (1983) A substance P antagonist inhibits vagally-induced increase in vascular permeability and bronchial smooth muscle contraction in the guinea pig. Proc Natl Acad Sci USA 80:1120–1124

Lygren I, Revhaug A, Burhol PG, Giercksky KE, Jenssen TG (1984) Vasoactive intestinal polypeptide and somatostatin in leucocytes. Scand J Clin Lab Invest 44:347–351

Marchetti B, Guarcello V, Morale MC, Bartoloni G, Farinella Z, Cordaro S, Scapagnini U (1989) Luteinizing hormone-releasing hormone-binding sites in the rat thymus: characteristics and biological function. Endocrinology 125:1025–1036

Marchetti B, Maier CC, LeBoeuf RD, Blalock JE (1990) Luteinizing hormone-releasing hormone gene expression in the thymus. Annual meeting of the society for Neuroscience, 28 Oct–2 Nov, 1990, St Louis, Missouri

Mathews PM, Froelich CJ, Sibbitt WL, Bankhurst AD (1983) Enhancement of natural cytotoxicity by β-endorphin. J Immunol 130:1658–1662

McIlhinney RAJ, Schulster D (1975) Studies on the binding of ^{125}I-labelled corticotropin to isolated rat adrenocortical cells. J Endocrinol 64:175–184

Merrill JE, Kutsunai S, Mohlstrom C, Hofman F, Groopman J, Golde DW (1984) Proliferation of astroglia and oligodendroglia in response to human T-cell-derived factors. Science 224: 1428–1430

Moore TC (1984) Modification of lymphocyte traffic by vasoactive neurotransmitter substance. Immunology 52:511–518

Oates EL, Allaway GP, Armstrong GR, Boyajian RA, Kehrl JH, Prabhakar BS (1988) Human lymphocytes produce pro-opiomelanocortin gene-related transcripts. J Biol Chem 263: 10041–10044

Oleson DR, Johnson DR (1988) Regulation of human natural cytotoxicity by enkephalins and selective opiate agonists. Brain Behav Immun 2:171–186

Ottaway CA (1984) In vitro alteration of receptors for vasoactive intestinal peptide changes the in vivo localization of mouse T-cells. J Exp Med 160: 1054–1069

Ottaway CA, Greenberg GR (1984) Interaction of vasoactive intestinal peptide with mouse lymphocytes: specific binding and the modulation of mitogen responses. J Immunol 132:417–423

Pawlikowski M, Stepien H, Kunert-Radek J, Schally AV (1985) Effect of somatostatin on the proliferation of mouse spleen lymphocytes in vitro. Biochem Biophys Res Commun 129:52–55

Pawlikowski M, Zelazowski P, Dohler KD, Stepien H (1988) Effects of two neuropeptides: Somatoliberin (GHRH) and corticoliberin (CRF) on human lymphocyte natural killer activity. Brain Behav Immun 2:50–56

Payan DG, Brewster DR, Goetzl EJ (1983) Specific stimulation of human T-lymphocytes by substance P. J Immunol 131:1613–1615

Payan DG, Brewster DR, Missirian-Bastian A, Goetzl EJ (1984a) Substance P recognition by a subset of human T-lymphocytes. J Clin Invest 74:1532–1539

Payan DG, Hess CA, Goetzl EJ (1984b) Inhibition by somatostatin of the proliferation of T-lymphocytes and Molt-4 lymphoblasts. Cell Immunol 84:433–438

Payan DG, Levine JD, Goetzl EJ (1984c) Modulation of immunity and hypersensitivity by sensory neuropeptides. J Immunol 132:1601–1604

Piotrowski W, Mead M, Foreman JC (1987) Action of the SP2-11 and SP3-11 fragments of substance P on rat peritoneal mast T-cells. Agents Actions 20: 178–180

Rivier CL, Plotsky PM (1986) Mediation by corticotropin-releasing factor of adenohypophysial hormone secretion. Annu Rev Physiol 48:475–494

Rola-Pleszczynski M, Bulduc D, St Pierre A (1985) The effects of VIP on human NK cell function. J Immunol 135:2659–2673

Ruff MR, Wahl SM, Pert CB (1985) Substance P receptor-mediated chemotaxis of human monocytes. Peptides 6:107–111

Sasaki A, Shinkawa O, Margioris AN, Liotta AS, Sato S, Murakami O, Go M, Shimizu Y, Hanew K, Yoshinaga K (1987) Immunoreactive corticotropin-releasing hormone in human plasma during pregnancy, labor, and delivery. J Clin Endocrinol Metab 64:224–229

Sasaki A, Shuichi S, Shigeru Y, Hanew K, Miru Y, Yoshinaga K (1989) Multiple forms of immunoreactive growth hormone-releasing hormone in human plasma, hypothalamus, and tumor tissues. J Clin Endocrinol Metab 68:180–185

Shanahan F, Denburg JA, Fox J, Bienenstock J, Befus D (1985) Mast cell heterogeneity: effects of neuroenteric peptides on histamine release. J Immunol 135:1331–1337

Shibasaki T, Odagiri E, Shizume K, Rainey N (1982) Corticotropin-releasing factor-like activity in human placental extracts. J Clin Endocrinol Metab 55:384–386

Shibasaki T, Kiyosawa Y, Masuda A, Nakahara M, Imaki T, Wakabayashi I, Demura H, Shizume K, Ling N (1984) Distribution of growth hormone-releasing hormone-like immunoreactivity in human tissue extracts. J Clin Endocrinol Metab 59:263–268

Singh VK (1989) Stimulatory effect of corticotropin releasing neurohormone on human lymphocyte proliferation and interleukin-2 receptor expression. J Neuroimmunol 23:257–262

Smith EM, Blalock JE (1981) Human lymphocyte production of ACTH and endorphin-like substances: association with leukocyte interferon. Proc Natl Acad Sci USA 78:7530–7534

Smith EM, Meyer WJ, Blalock JE (1982) Virus induced increases in corticosterone in hypophysectomy mice: a possible lymphoid-adrenal axis. Science 218:1311–1313

Smith EM, Phan M, Coppenhaver D, Kruger TE, Blalock JE (1983) Human lymphocyte production of immunoreactive thyrotropin. Proc Natl Acad Sci USA 80:6010–6013

Smith EM, Morrill AC, Meyer WJ, Blalock JE (1986) Corticotropin releasing factor induction of leukocyte-derived immunoreactive ACTH and endorphins. Nature 322:881–882

Smith EM, Galin FS, LeBoeuf RD, Copenhaver DH, Harbour DV, Blalock JE (1990) Nucleotide and amino acid sequence of lymphocyte-derived corticotropin: endotoxin induction of truncated peptide. Proc Natl Acad Sci USA 87:1057–1060

Stanisz AM, Befus D, Bienenstock J (1986) Differential effects of vasoactive intestinal peptide, substance P, and somatostatin on immunoglobulin synthesis and proliferations by lymphocytes from Peyer's patches, mesenteric lymph nodes, and spleen. J Immunol 136:152–156

Stanisz AM, Scicchitano R, Payan DG, Bienenstock J (1987a) In vitro studies of immunoregulation of substance P and somatostatin. Ann NY Acad Sci 496:217–225

Stanisz AM, Scicchitano R, Dazin P, Bienenstock J, Payan DG (1987b) Distribution of substance P receptors on murine spleen and Peyer's patch T- and B-cells. J Immunol 139:749–754

Stephanou A, Jessop DS, Knight RA, Lightman SL (1990) Corticotropin-releasing factor-like immunoreactivity and mRNA in human leukocytes. Brain Behav Immun 4:67–73

Theoharides TC, Douglas WW (1981) Mast cell histamine secretion in response to somatostatin analogues: structural considerations. Eur J Pharmacol 73:131–136

Van Epps D, Saland L (1984) β-Endorphin and Met-enkephalin stimulate human peripheral blood mononuclear cell chemotaxis. J Immunol 132:3046–3053

Weigent DA, Blalock JE (1987) Interactions between the neuroendocrine and immune systems: common hormones and receptors. Immunol Rev 100:79–108

Weigent DA, Blalock JE (1990) Immunoreactive growth hormone-releasing hormone in rat leukocytes. J Neuroimmunol 29:1–13

Weigent DA, Baxter JB, Wear WE, Smith LR, Bost KL, Blalock JE (1988) Production of immunoreactive growth hormone by mononuclear leukocytes. FASEB J 2:2812–2818

Weinstock JV, Blum AM (1990) Release of substance P by granuloma eosinophils in response to secretagogues in murine Schistosomiasis mansoni. Cell Immunol 125:380–385

Wenger GD, O'Dorisio MS (1990) Vasoactive intestinal peptide: messenger in a neuroimmune axis. Ann NY Acad Sci 594:104–119

Westley HJ, Kleiss AJ, Kelley KW, Wong PKY, Yuen P-H (1986) Newcastle's disease virus-infected splenocytes express the pro-opiomelanocortin gene. J Exp Med 163:1589–1594

Woloski BMRNJ, Smith EM, Meyer WJ III, Fuller GM, Blalock JE (1985) Corticotropin-releasing activity of monokines. Science 23:1035–1037

Yasuda N, Greer MA, Azizawa T (1982) Corticotropin-releasing factor. Endocr Rev 3: 123

Zelazowski P, Dohler KD, Stepien H, Pawlikowski M (1989) Effect of growth hormone releasing hormone on human peripheral blood leukocyte chemotaxis and migration in normal subjects. Neuroendocrinology 50:236

Corticotropin and Immunoregulation

E. M. Smith

Introduction

Corticotropin (ACTH) is a neuropeptide first found in the pituitary gland and well known for its ability to stimulate adrenal steroidogenesis. Recent findings have shown ACTH to be synthesized in various tissues other than the pituitary. It has been identified in several regions of the brain (Krieger et al. 1977; Liotta and Krieger 1983), reproductive tissues (Margioris et al. 1983) including the placenta (Liotta et al. 1977), and immune tissues (Smith and Blalock 1981; Smith and Johnson 1988; Smith et al. 1991). Furthermore, ACTH has been demonstrated in the nervous tissue and hemolymph of invertebrates (Smith et al. 1991, for review). There is evidence suggesting that parasite-derived ACTH inactivates certain host defenses (Duvaux-Miret et al. 1992).

The information summarized in this chapter makes a strong case for the conclusion that one of the several important roles of ACTH is that of regulating immunobiological activities. A consideration of the possible sources and molecular species of ACTH may be the discussion of its function as an immunomodulator.

Pituitary ACTH

ACTH is coproduced, along with endorphins and α-melanocyte stimulating hormone (α-MSH) from the large polyprotein pro-opiomelanocortin (POMC). The POMC gene is a characteristically split eukaryotic gene. It consists of three exons divided by two large intervening sequences (Chang et al. 1980). Exon 1 codes for an untranslated region as does the first part of exon 2. The remainder of the second exon codes for the signal sequence. Exon 3 codes for the POMC polyprotein. At the protein level, differential processing of POMC results in multiple species of ACTH and other active peptides such as the endorphins. Full-length ACTH consists of 39 amino acids. The amino terminal (10 residues)

Department of Psychiatry and Behavioral Sciences, University of Texas Medical Branch, Galveston TX 77550, USA

Scharrer et al. (Eds.)
Neuropeptides and Immunoregulation

is needed for full steroidogenic activity and has been highly conserved during evolution. Conversely, the sequence of the 15 carboxyl terminal amino acids is species specific (Li 1972). Posttranslational modification of POMC varies with the different sites of synthesis. In the anterior pituitary the major products are $ACTH_{1-39}$, β-lipotropin, and *N*-POMC (Krieger 1983). In species that possess an intermediate pituitary the major products are α-MSH and β-endorphin. The proteolytic processing occurs at paired basic amino acid residues. Not all of these sites appear to be susceptible to hydrolysis in the anterior pituitary; in the intermediate lobe other sites of cleavage are used.

Additional posttranslational modifications include amidation and acetylation at the carboxyl and amino terminal residues, respectively. These modifications are important because they greatly affect the molecules's activity and stability. For instance, amidated α-MSH has virtually no ACTH activity (Hirsch and O'Donohue 1986). Also, acetylation of β-endorphin diminishes its opiate binding activity (Akil et al. 1981). Thus, the combination of proteolytic cleavage and modifications of the terminal groups permits one POMC gene to be the source of multiple active products having a variety of functions.

Extrapituitary ACTH

ACTH has been identified in the brains of normal and hypophysectomized rats (Krieger et al. 1977). The same group (Liotta et al. 1977) also reported its presence in human placenta and demonstrated that it is synthesized there de novo. Later, ACTH was demonstrated in the gastrointestinal tract (Larsson 1981; Tanaka et al. 1982) and in the testis (Margioris et al. 1983). In the brain, ACTH is located in the hypothalamus as well as in cells and axons of other regions such as the hippocampus and cortex (Liotta and Krieger 1983; Smith and Founder 1988). Many of these studies determined only ACTH and POMC immunoreactivity, but some characterized the peptides biochemically, and more recent contributions have identified POMC mRNA in these tissues (Lacaze-Masmonteil et al. 1987). As in the pituitary, α-MSH and β-endorphin are also frequently found in association with ACTH.

Little is known about the regulation of ACTH production in these extrapituitary tissues. Anterior pituitary ACTH is induced by corticotropin-releasing factor (CRF), vasopressin, and α-adrenergic agents and inhibited by glucocorticoids (Krieger 1983). In contrast, brain ACTH levels appear to be constant, failing to change in response to prototypical releasing hormones, stress, or removal of adrenal steroids (O'Donohue et al. 1979). Placental ACTH production also does not respond to glucocorticoid administration (Liotta et al. 1977).

The specific role of ACTH in these extrapituitary tissues has yet to be determined. Krieger (1983) has suggested some possible functions such as in sexual and learning behavior or stimulation of Sertoli cell growth. Specific activities may depend on the posttranslational modifications of the peptides (many are acetylated) and the presence of cofactors (Strand et al. 1991). Interestingly, more seems to be known about ACTH action in the immune system than in other extrapituitary sites.

ACTH Production in the Immune System

Aside from the role played by ACTH in the mediation of neuroendocrine signals to the immune system, this peptide released from immunoactive cells is instrumental in the system's autoregulatory activities. The presence of immunoactive ACTH in human leukocytes was reported by Blalock and Smith in 1980 (see also Scharrer and Stefano, this volume).

Structurally, the POMC-derived peptides found in these cells are the same as those of the pituitary (Smith et al. 1990a). Recent evidence suggests that the POMC mRNA in immune cells is a truncated version of pituitary POMC mRNA (Galin et al. 1990). This abbreviated form, however, still contains the third exon sequence which codes for ACTH and β-lipotropin.

ACTH and β-endorphin are produced constitutively by murine splenic macrophages (Lolait et al. 1984) and mast cells (DiAugustine et al. 1980) but generally need to be induced in lymphocytes (Blalock and Smith 1980; Smith and Blalock 1981; Smith et al. for review). In parallel with the similarities in structure, regulation of production from POMC in leukocytes resembles that in the pituitary (Blalock and Smith 1982; Smith et al. 1986). CRF the principal inducer of pituitary ACTH (Rivier et al. 1983), also stimulates leukocyte ACTH production and release (Smith et al. 1986). This has been confirmed by Kavelaars et al. (1989) who expanded the finding to show that CRF acts through stimulating interleukin-1 (IL-1) in macrophages. Webster and DeSouza (1988); Webster et al. (1989) previously found concentrated binding of CRF to macrophage-rich areas of rat spleens. Others reported B-cell (McGillis et al. 1889) and T-Cell (Singh 1989) activation by CRF. Thus, there appears to be at least one more mechanism for CRF to stimulate leukocyte production of ACTH.

Newcastle disease virus (NDV) was the first inducer of leukocyte ACTH reported (Blalock and Smith 1980; Smith and Blalock 1981; Westly et al. 1986). Other nonlytic viruses also induce ACTH. Epstein-Barr virus transforms B-cells (Oates et al. 1988, 1990), and human immunodeficiency virus (HIV) infected T-cells also produce ACTH and MSH (Smith et al. 1992). Inactive virus preparations such as influenza virus vaccine and synthetic double stranded RNA which mimics a viral RNA replicative intermediate also induce lymphoid ACTH production (Smith et al., unpublished).

The B-cell mitogen bacterial lipopolysaccharide (LPS), is another potent inducer of ACTH production by B-lymphocytes, (Harbour-McMenamin et al. 1985). In contrast to CRF- or NDV-induced ACTH, that induced by LPS is truncated and is approximately the size of $ACTH_{1-24}$ (Harbour et al. 1987). Thus, within the immune system there is alternate processing of POMC. Since these inducers can act on the same cell (i.e., NDV, CRF, and LPS all act on B-Cells), this processing is probably a result of different pathways (and enzymes) being activated.

Undoubtedly, other inducers will be found. Thymopentin, the active pentapeptide of thympoietin, is a recent addition to the list of inducers (Buzzetti et al. 1989). Consequently, in assessing the concentrations necessary for effects of ACTH on the immune system, it is relevant that the peptide is produced by many tissues and cells, including those of the immune system.

Vertebrate tissues expressing ACTH are the following adapted from Krieger 1983, and reproduced with permission from Smith et al. 1991:

- Brain
- Placenta
- Pituitary
- Reproductive tract
  - Testis
  - Vas deferens
  - Epididymis
  - Seminal vesicles
  - Ovary
- Gastrointestinal tract
  - Stomach
  - Pancreas
  - Intestine
- Lung
- Immune system
  - Lymphocytes (B,T)
  - Macrophages
  - Granulocytes

ACTH Immunomodulation

In understanding the immunomodulatory activity of ACTH it is necessary to consider potential indirect actions of the neuropeptide. There are at least two ways by which ACTH acts indirectly. One is through induction of steroids (Munck et al. 1984), and the other is through secondary transformation into MSH (Smith et al. 1992), which is also a powerful immunomodulator (Van Epps and Mason 1990; Van Epps, this volume). In the past , the ACTH effects on the immune system were thought to be largely indirect, mediated through induction of corticosteroid hormones (see Berczi 1986, for review). Corticosteroids are certainly important modulators of immune function. They are potent immunosuppressive agents at high doses, yet in vitro they are required at low doses for maximal immune responsiveness. MSH is also potently immunosuppressive, as covered in detail elsewhere in this volume (Van Epps). Nonetheless, the fact that ACTH, added in vitro to leukocyte cultures, rapidly affects certain responses clearly demonstrates that ACTH has inherent and direct effects.

Inhibition of antibody production was the first immunological effect attributable to ACTH (Johnson et al. 1982). It was found to suppress antibody production in an in vitro plaque-forming cell assay against two antigens, sheep red blood cells and dinitrophenol. Munn and Lum (1989) also found that ACTH inhibits specific antibody synthesis in response to a defined antigen, tetanus toxoid. However, when higher concentrations of ACTH were used (10^{-9}, 10^{-11} versus 10^{-13}, 10^{-17} M) the production of antibody to the tetanus toxoid was actually enhanced. Conversely, Bost et al. (1990) found that ACTH in picomolar amounts enhances a murine B-cell line to secrete IgM, while micromolar amounts inhibit the secretion.

Several related findings on the effect of ACTH on B-lymphocytes suggest possible mechanisms for these seemingly conflicting results. Alvarez-Mon et al. (1985) found that ACTH enhances B-cell growth and differentiation in conjunction with a B-cell growth factor or IL-2. Similarly, a recent report by Brooks (1990) demonstrated that ACTH functions as a late-acting B-cell growth factor and synergizes with IL-5, a known B-cell growth factor. Little is known about expression of ACTH receptors on B-cells at different stages of maturation. The differences between the responses of the cell lines and fresh peripheral blood lymphocytes or splenocytes might be due to differences in cell type or the presence of helper cells. In this regard, ACTH has also been reported to inhibit T-lymphocyte proliferation in response to a mitogen (Heijnen et al. 1987). Thus, ACTH may affect antibody synthesis at multiple levels, either directly by signals to the plasma cell or indirectly through altering cellular production of growth and differentiation factors.

Since cytokines play a major role in regulating immune responses such as antibody production, it is of interest that the production of several of these is altered by ACTH. Interferon-γ (IFN-γ) production by T-lymphocytes is inhibited (Johnson et al. 1984), as is IFN-γ activation of tumoricidal activity of macrophages (Koff and Dunegan 1985). However, the production of tumor necrosis factor-α (TNF-α), by adherent cells is induced by ACTH (Hughes and Smith 1990). Whereas, ACTH inhibits IFN-γ activation of macrophages, the combination of these two factors actually synergizes and enhances TNF-α production.

ACTH probably acts on most leukocytes, but T-lymphocytes seem particularly sensitive to its effects. Johnson et al. (1982) found that antibody suppression is greater when the response is directed against a T-lymphocyte dependent antigen. However, there was still 81% suppression when a T-independent antigen was used. Apparently, ACTH affects the B-cells, but maximal suppression occurs only when T-cell help is also altered. IFN-γ production is another T-cell function suppressed by ACTH (Johnson et al. 1984). Phorbol myristate, which replaces T-helper cell activity, failed to reverse the inhibition, thereby confirming that ACTH can act directly on T-cells. Suppression of lymphocyte proliferation in response to a T-cell mitogen, concanavalin A (con A), also supports a direct action of ACTH on T-cells (Heijnen et al. 1987).

The use of purified cell preparations and cell lines clearly shows that B-cells are directly affected by ACTH. Less specific but supportive is the finding that

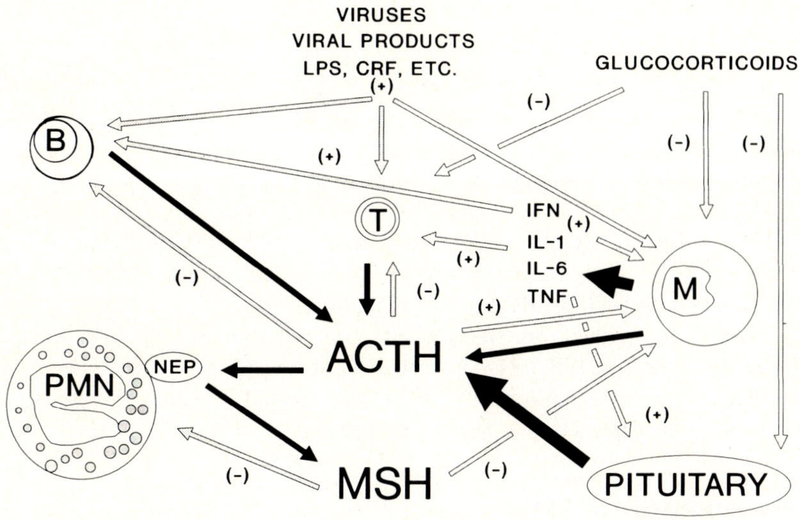

Fig. 1. Major interactions between the nervous and immune systems involving ACTH, other hormones, and cytokines. Sites of synthesis (*solid arrows*) and modulatory activities (*shaded arrows*). Enhancement or inhibition of activities indicated by plus and minus symbols, respectively. *B*, B-lymphocyte; *CRF*, corticotropin-releasing factor; *IFN*, interferon; *IL*, interleukin; *LPS*, bacterial lipopolysaccharide; *M*, macrophage/monocyte; *NEP*, neutral endopeptidase; *PMN*, polymorphonuclear leukocyte; *T*, T-lymphocyte; *TNF*, tumor necrosis factor

ACTH suppresses antibody production against a T-independent antigen, as discussed above (Johnson et al. 1982). Alvarez-Mon et al. (1985) used highly purified preparations of human tonsillar B-cells in their study of ACTH enhancement of growth and differentiation. Bost et al. (1987) demonstrated the presence of both ACTH and its receptor on a B-lymphocytic cell line (BCL_1). Brooks (1990) confirmed this using the 3B3 clone of this cell line and showing that ACTH functions as a late-acting growth factor synergizing with IL-5. Bost et al. (1990) also used a B-cell line, CH12.LX.C4.5F5, in their study of the effects of ACTH on IgM secretion.

Monocytes and macrophages could be involved in ACTH inhibition of antibody production (Johnson et al. 1984) since they produce IL-1 and also respond to ACTH. Activation of macrophage tumoricidal activity by IFN-γ is inhibited by ACTH (Koff and Dinegan 1985). This could possibly be mediated through inhibition of TNF production, but Hughes and Smith (1990) found that ACTH actually induces macrophage cultures to produce TNF. IL-1 is usually coproduced with TNF and IL-6, and these cytokines in turn stimulate ACTH production (see Hughes and Chin, this volume). As depicted in Fig. 1, the cytokines interact at multiple points and thus implicate the macrophage/monocytic cells as key elements in these responses.

Action of ACTH

The results obtained from the study on the effects of neuropeptides on the immune system vary, especially those with regard to ACTH. Possible reasons for this variability range from the use of inactive peptide preparations and contamination with endotoxin to the very real possibility of enzymatic breakdown of the neuropeptide (Smith et al. 1992; Turner et al., this volume). Heijnen et al. (1987) noted that some variability is due to the individual donors. In 65% of donors ACTH inhibited lymphocyte proliferation induced by con A, whereas 23% showed a positive effect, and 12% did not react.

There are at least three factors influencing the mode of action of ACTH in the immune system: specific effects dependent upon the molecular species of ACTH, the presence of the respective receptors on the target cells, and the activation of intracellular target systems by the receptors.

Processing of ACTH

The primary factor determining the effects of ACTH is the probably posttranslational processing of its polyprotein precursor. POMC is not generally released, and it is inactive until it has been processed. The first 18 residues ($ACTH_{1-18}$) are required for steroidogenic activity. Some of the studies have revealed differences in the forms in which ACTH is immunomodulatory. In its effects on IFN-γ production, only full-length $ACTH_{1-39}$ is inhibitory (Johnson et al. 1984). This contrasts with its steroidogenic activity which resides in the first 18 residues ($ACTH_{1-18}$) and suggests that breakdown into MSH is not a factor in inhibiting in vitro antibody production. B-cell growth and differentiation are enhanced by a synthetic $ACTH_{1-24}$ as effectively as with natural, full-length ACTH (Alvarez-Mon et al. 1985). Also, only full-length ACTH is effective on TNF induction in adherent cells (Hughes and Smith 1990).

Since MSH is also a peptide with immunomodulating activity (Van Epps, this volume) subsequent or secondary processing of ACTH to MSH must be considered. Van Epps and Mason (1990) have noted that MSH is a more potent inhibitor of polymorphonuclear leukocyte migration than ACTH and suggest that ACTH may be processed to MSH in the immune system. In the case of human granulocytes and *Mytilus* immunocytes this suggestion has recently been found to be correct (Smith et al. 1992). Neutral endopeptidase (NEP 24.11) is present on these cells (Shipp et al. 1990; Turner et al., this volume), and ACTH is much slower than MSH in inhibiting spontaneous activation of both cell types. ACTH requires over 2 h whereas MSH is effective in 20 min. This time period suffices to process ACTH to MSH. Phosphoramidon, a specific inhibitor of NEP, blocks ACTH inhibition of cellular activation and thereby provides further support for this concept. Addition of ACTH to granulocytes and monitoring for ACTH and MSH show a consistent decrease in ACTH with rising MSH levels, which can be slowed down by phosphoramidon.

NEP is present in the liver and, known as CD10, on many lymphoid cells (Turner et al., this volume). Also, the expression of NEP can be modulated (Shipp et al. 1990), and it can be expected that these mechanisms represent local means of regulating ACTH immunomodulatory properties.

Receptors

An indication that ACTH has direct and specific effects is the presence of specific leukocyte receptors coupled to intracellular pathways. Initially, Johnson et al. (1982) reported high-affinity binding to murine splenocytes along with ACTH inhibition of antibody production. Smith et al. (1987) found that mononuclear cells of human peripheral blood also possess high-affinity ACTH binding sites, and that the functioning of these lymphoid "receptors" correlates with adrenal ACTH receptors in a case of ACTH insufficiency syndrome. Bost et al. (1987) reported that the murine B-lymphocytic cell line BCL_1 expressed ACTH receptors. Johnson et al. (1988) and then Clarke and Bost (1989) reported that murine lymphoid ACTH receptors can be upregulated with con A.

It appears certain that lymphocytes and probably macrophages have ACTH receptors. PMNs probably have MSH receptors, a suggestion based on the relative efficacy of MSH versus ACTH (Van Epps and Mason 1990; Smith et al. 1992). Currently there is no indication that macrophages respond to MSH. This is suggested indirectly by the failure of MSH to affect IFN-γ induction (Johnson et al. 1984) and TNF induction by a truncated form of ACTH, $ACTH_{1-24}$ (Hughes and Smith 1990).

Several radioligand binding studies have been performed to suggest which major lymphoid cell types express ACTH receptors. Johnson et al. (1982) were the first to report that ACTH binds to lymphoid cells. Intact murine splenocytes were found to have high- and lower-affinity binding sites. Smith et al. (1987) reported ACTH receptors of both high and lower affinity to be present on mononuclear cells of human peripheral blood. Of note is the fact that there appears to be a correlation between lack of high-affinity binding on leukocytes and defective adrenal response to ACTH in a case of ACTH insufficiency syndrome.

Johnson (1989) used a combination of immunofluorescence and radioligand binding data to identify murine leukocyte populations that bear ACTH receptors. Approximately 50% of B-cells and monocyte/macrophage cells plus less than 20% of mature T-cells seem to have the receptor. Thymocytes are essentially devoid of ACTH receptors, unless stimulated by a T-cell mitogen such as con A. Clarke and Bost (1989) reported similar results in rat splenocytes. The presence of high- and lower affinity binding sites is a consistent finding even when a cell line (BCL_1) or purified receptors are examined (Bost et al. 1987). Jaramillo et al. (unpublished) reexamined the BCL_1 and human mononuclear cells using an improved binding assay with a very low level of nonspecific binding. High- and lower affinity binding sites were found in both cell types, but the relative affinities of these sites were reduced by two orders of magnitude as compared to the earlier results.

Intracellular Mechanisms of ACTH

Another functional link that shows specificity is activation of intracellular signal pathways. Stimulation of adrenal steroidogenesis by ACTH is accompanied by activation of adenylate cyclase (Ways et al. 1976). Because of the presence of high- and low affinity binding sites on adrenal cells and increased cAMP levels usually associated only with high concentrations of ACTH, a solid cause-effect relationship has not been established for this messenger system. Johnson et al. (1988) have demonstrated that cAMP increases in dissociated murine splenocytes and a cultured T-cell line treated with ACTH. In a comparison between two human T-cell lymphoma cell lines, S49A and Molt 4 cells, cAMP was induced by ACTH only in the former which expressed the ACTH receptor. Clarke and Bost (1989) also found cAMP to be induced in rat splenocytes by ACTH. Kavelaars et al. (1988) detected another possible second messenger pathway, mediated by intracellular calcium. They reported that ACTH at 0.1 n*M* enhances the cytosolic free calcium in T-cells activated by con A or RIV_9. ACTH had no effect on baseline free calcium concentrations in these studies.

Although comparatively little is known concerning the intracellular messenger systems mediating ACTH effects on lymphoid cells, this may be the most important level for determining its action. Lymphocytes possess receptors for many cytokines and neuropeptides. Since the cells are constantly exposed to these factors in the serum, some discrimination or integration at the extra- or intracellular levels must occur. An understanding of a cell's response to multiple signals in the milieu will be the key to knowledge of the effect of ACTH on the immune system.

Comparative Aspects of the Role of ACTH in Immunomodulation

The elucidation of the immunomodulatory activities of ACTH and other neuropeptides has made considerable progress by recent investigations in higher invertebrates. ACTH has been reported to be present in representatives of most phyla, including protozoans. As in vertebrates, this compound is found in neuroendocrine as well as immunoactive structures. Several of these studies have been carried out by immunocytochemical analysis. For example, Boer et al. (1979) reported ACTH reactivity in two electrically coupled gaint neurons of the pond snail *Lymnaea stagnalis*. A material resembling vertebrate ACTH and MSH was found in the neuroendocrine system of the insect *Leucophaea maderae* (Hansen et al. 1986). Ottaviani et al. (1990) demonstrated ACTH and β-endorphin in the hemolymph and hemocytes of the freshwater snail *Planorbarius corneus*. This study along with the results on *Mytilus edulis* discussed below (Smith et al. 1990b) was the first to report on ACTH associated with the invertebrate immune system.

ACTH has been found in the following invertebrates:

Arthropoda
- *Periplaneta americana* (Schols et al. 1987)
- *Leucophaea maderae* (Hansen et al. 1986)
- *Locusta migratoria* (Rafaeli et al. 1987)

Aschelminthes
- *Goodeyus ulmi* (Leach et al. 1987)

Mollusca
- *Mytilus edulis* (Smith et al. 1990)
- *Lymnaea stagnalis* (Boer et al. 1979)
- *Planorbarius corneus* (Ottaviani et al. 1990)

Protozoa
- *Tetrahymena pyriformis* (LeRoith et al. 1982)
- *Schistosoma mansoni* (Duvaux-Miret and Capron 1991)

As in vertebrates, the function of ACTH in the nervous system is virtually unknown. An interesting report by Rafaeli et al. (1987) demonstrates an immunological cross reactivity between ACTH and the diuretic hormone of locusts; ACTH stimulated fluid secretion and cAMP secretion in locust Malpighian tubules. It seems likely that ACTH has endocrine and neurotransmitter functions in many organisms.

It is not too surprising to find ACTH and POMC products in invertebrate immune cells (Ottoviani et al. 1991; Smith et al. 1991) in view of the results obtained in *Mytilus edulis* by Stefano et al. (1989). These authors demonstrated the production of opioid peptides by, and their action on, hemocytes of this mollusc which resemble cells of the granulocyte/monocyte lineage of vertebrates (Lolait et al. 1984).

We have detected irACTH by radioimmunoassay in hemolymph of *Mytilus edulis* and have preliminarily shown it to be biologically active and antigenically identical with ACTH standards (Smith et al. 1990b). A possible source of this irACTH is the immunocyte, as seen in vertebrates (Smith et al. 1991, for review) and in the snail *Planorbarius* (Ottaviani et al. 1990). The other obvious possibility is that some or all of the irACTH in hemolymph comes from the nervous system.

The role of ACTH in invertebrate hemolymph may be immunomodulation in addition to some other signal function, as suggested above. When ACTH and MSH were assessed for the ability to alter immunocyte conformation and motility of *M. edulis* (Fig. 2), results similar to those in human granulocytes were obtained (Fig. 3; Stefano et al. 1991; Smith et al. 1992). ACTH itself does not appear to alter the activity, i.e., the conformational state of inactive or active hemocytes in short-term (20 min) assays, whereas both α- and β-MSH induced active ameboid hemocytes to become rounded-inactive in a dose-dependent fashion (Fig. 2). α-MSH also inactivates ameboid hemocytes stimulated

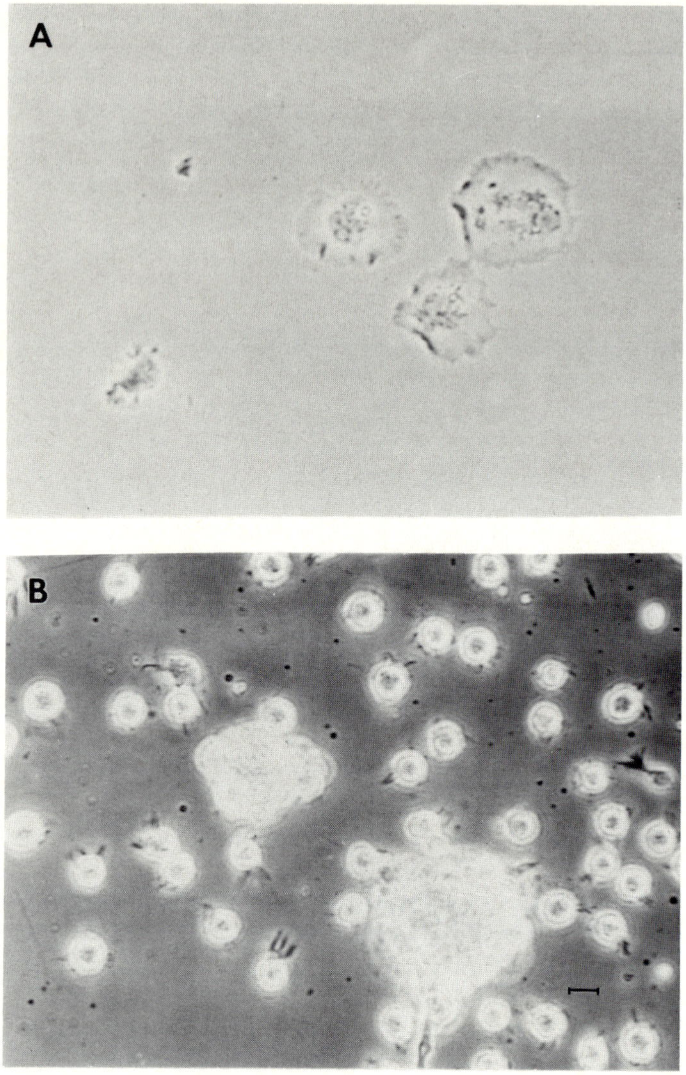

Fig. 2A, B. Videomicrographs of spontaneously active Mytilus immunocytes (**A**) and those treated for 30 min with 10^{-8} *M* α-MSH. (**B**) *Bar*, (lower right corner, **B**), 10 μm

with β-endorphin or TNF. As in human granulocytes, ACTH inactivates the immunocytes after 4 h of incubation whereas the effect of α-MSH occurs in minutes (Fig. 3). The effect of ACTH is blocked by phosphoramidon. Therefore it is likely that the major inhibitory activity on *Mytilus* immunocytes is due to MSH following ACTH cleavage by NEP.

ACTH has been reported to enhance immunocyte migration and phagocytic activity of cells of the snail *Planorbarius corneus* (Ottoviani et al. 1991). The

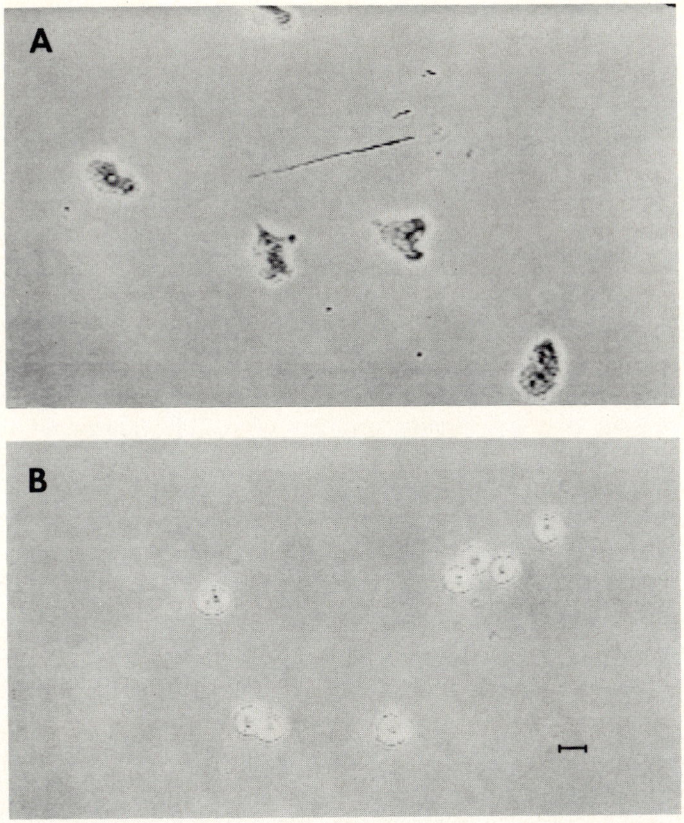

Fig. 3A, B. Videomicrographs of spontaneously active human granulocytes (**A**) and those treated for 20 min with 10^{-8} M α-MSH (**B**), *Bar*, (lower right corner, **B**), 10 μm

kinetics of the phagocytosis shows a dramatic jump in activity after 2 h, which, based on the discussion above, suggests that processing may also occur in this system, and that MSH may be a mediator of the effect. Another effect of ACTH on *Planorbarius* immunocytes reported by Ottoviani et al. (1991) is the release of biogenic amines; exposure of the hemocytes to ACTH caused a reduction in the cellular contents of norepinephrine, epinephrine, and dopamine with a concomitant rise in the hemolymph level of these amines.

There clearly appears to be some role for ACTH and MSH in regulating the functions of invertebrate immunocytes.

Biomedical Implications of ACTH Immunomodulation

The new insights gained on the immunosuppressive effects of ACTH are of more than academic interest. Two clinical examples will serve to make this point.

Humun Immunodeficiency Virus Infection

A hallmark of the acquired immune-deficiency syndrome (AIDS) is the extent of the systemic effects observed when relatively few cells are actually infected by HIV (Harper et al. 1986). Activation of the hypothalamic-hypophysial-adrenal axis and the resultant release of corticosteroid hormones have been reported in early stages of HIV infection (Centers for Disease Control stages II and III) (Verges et al. 1989). However, no direct relationship was established between this rise in cortisol and the course of the disease.

A more direct role of ACTH has been suggested by in vitro studies demonstrating that a cell line infected from 15 to 58 days with the HIV virus produces consistent levels of ACTH, MSH, and other POMC-derived peptides (Fig. 4, Smith et al. 1992). The same study provided evidence that the MSH present is a conversion product of ACTH, presumed to be processed by neutral endopeptidase. The induction of ACTH by HIV occurs much more slowly than that by NDV, requiring 3–4 weeks to reach a significant level. This may explain why Oates et al. (1988) did not see a rise in POMC mRNA levels in lymphocytes that had been infected with HIV for only 48 h. This delay in the production of ACTH seems to be directly related to the virus, as there is some correspondence between the virulence of the viral strain and the speed of ACTH production (Hashemi et al., unpublished). Hashemi et al. (1992) have examined the effects on ACTH production of three isolates of HIV-1 in peripheral

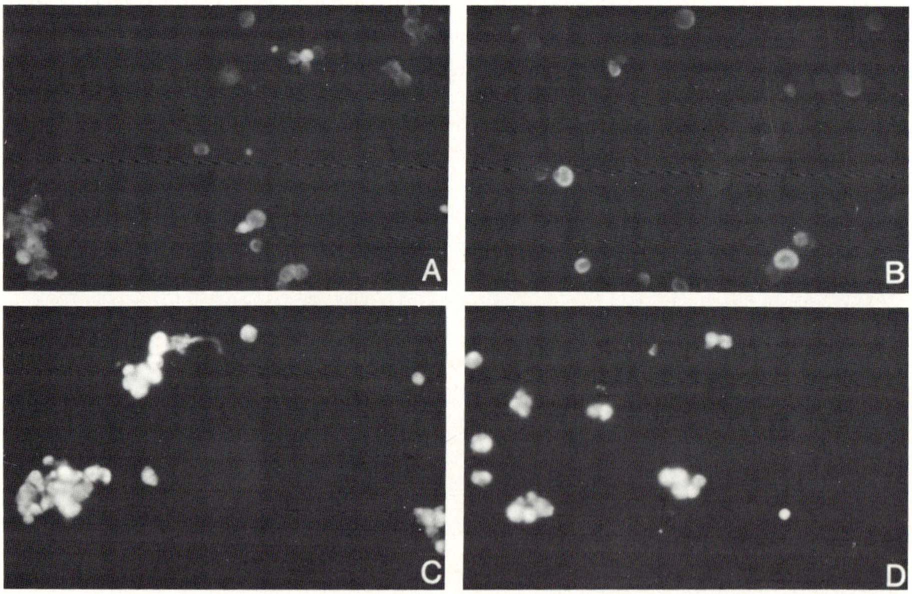

Fig. 4A–D. Infected cells stained by immunofluorescence with normal rabbit serum 45 days after infection (**A**) anti-ACTH 25 days after infection (**B**), anti-ACTH 45 days after infection (**C**), and anti-p24 stained 45 days after infection (**D**). (Reproduced with permission from Smith et al. 1992)

blood lymphocytes and several T-cell lines. In all cells tested, ACTH production was correlated with the production of the viral capsid antigen p24. In H9 cells production of ACTH could be detected as early as 7 days, and the maximum number of producing cells was observed 20–30 days after the infection. Furthermore, the virus is not required to be infectious to stimulate ACTH production. Ultraviolet light inactivated virus or the major envelope glycoprotein gp120 initiates the response (Hashemi et al., unpublished).

These in vitro results are in line with recent studies on ACTH and MSH in AIDS patients. Catania et al. (1992) reported that MSH levels are elevated in these patients. Of particular interest is the finding that their levels of ACTH and MSH are inversely related. Thus, the cleavage of MSH from ACTH by neutral endopeptidase, surmised by Smith et al. (1992) in their in vitro experiments, appears to occur also in vivo. Another interesting findng of Catania et al. was a positive relationship among circulating ACTH, IL-6, and fever in their group of AIDS patients ($p < 0.01$). Thus, the study of AIDS confirms the concept of an immune-neuroendocrine network, the disturbance of which contributes to the clinical features of this syndrome.

Immunosuppression in Hosts by the Parasite's ACTH in Shistosomiasis

The parallel between the immunobiological roles of ACTH in invertebrate and human immunocytes is clear, and it seems to have functional implications beyond that of tracing the evolution of these systems. Mimicry of the host's antigens is a scheme utilized by parasites to avoid detection by the host's immune system. A special case of this scheme is schistosomiasis, where the parasites synthesize signal molecules resembling those of the host, apparently to escape the host's immune responses by suppression rather than camouflage (Duvaux–Miret and Capron 1991; Duvaux–Miret et al. 1992). POMC expression by the parasite *Schistosoma mansoni* results in the production of POMC-related peptides, i.e., β-endorphin, α-MSH in most stages of the life cycle of the worm. Adult worms and cercariae have the highest levels of the neuropeptides. ACTH and MSH inactivate immunocytes of both definitive (human, hamster) and intermediate (snail) hosts (Duvaux-Miret et al. 1992). Immunocytes of infected snails were found to be inactive, and this state could be reversed with antisera to ACTH and MSH. The obvious implication of these findings is that the parasite uses the same signal molecules as those of the hosts to compromise defenses or enhance their infection. It is an advantage made possible by the long evolutionary history of these molecules.

Conclusions

The major conclusion to be drawn at this time is that ACTH, derived from several sources, participates in the operation of the immune system. Its apparent roles concern exchange of information with the neuroendorine system, as well as autoimmunoregulatory processes. As to the mode of operation of ACTH, recent evidence supports the concept that its immunosuppressive role is in part indirect, i.e., by giving rise to MSH (Smith et al. 1992) and glucocorticoids (Munck et al. 1984).

The various activities of ACTH/MSH must be viewed as part of a complex control system (Fig. 1) in which various other hormones and cytokines interact. Additional controlling factors are the concentration and pattern of delivery of messenger molecules (continuous, pulsatile, etc.), kinetics, microenvironment, and presence and number of specific receptors. As depicted in Fig. 1, the actions of ACTH/MSH in the immune system are the result of an integration of all these factors.

For these interactions to have been so conserved through evolution, there must be some fundamental role beneficial to the host that has yet to be fully determined. Under certain pathological conditions (virus infections, schistosomiasis), a rise in the level of circulating ACTH/MSH and its concomitant immunosuppressive effect (Smith et al. 1982: Dupont et al. 1984: Catania et al. 1992) appear to influence the immune response of the host. Therefore, it is likely that with further investigation additional functions will be identified and will make possible a broader definition of the role of ACTH in the system.

Acknowledgements. Recent studies from the author's laboratory have been supported by grants from the Office of Naval Research (N00014–89–J–1095). National Institutes of Health (DK 41034). and the Department of Psychiatry at the University of Texas Medical Branch.

References

Akil H, Young E, Watson SJ (1981) Opiate binding properties of naturally occurring N- and C-terminus modified beta-endorphins. Peptides 2:289–292

Alvarez-Mon M, Kehrl JH, Fauci AS (1985) A potential role for adrenocorticotropin in regulating human B-lymphocyte functions. J Immunol 135:3823–3826

Berczi I (1986) *Pituitary function and immunity.* CRC Press, Boca Raton

Blalock JE, Smith EM (1980) Human leukocyte interferon: structure and biological relatedness to adrenocorticotropic hormone and endorphins. Proc Natl Acad Sci USA 77:5972–5974

Blalock JE, Smith EM (1982) Human lymphocyte production of neuroendocrine hormone-related substances. In. Khan A, Hill NO, Dumonds DC (eds) *Human lymphokines.* Academic Press, New York, pp 323–332

Boer HH, Schot LPC, Roubos EW, ter Maat A, Lodder JC, Reichelt D (1979) ACTH-like immunoreactivity in two electrotonically coupled giant neurons in the pond snail *Lymnaea stagnalis.* Cell Tissue Res 202:231–240

Bost KL, Smith EM, Wear LB, Blalock JE (1987) Presence of ACTH and its receptor on a B-lymphocytic cell line: a possible autocrine function for a neuroendocrine hormone. J Biol Regul Homeost Agents 1:23–27

Bost KL, Clarke BL, Xu J, Kiyono H, McGhee JR, Pascual D (1990) Modulation of IgM secretion and H chain mRNA expression in CH12.LX.C4. 5F5 B-cells by adrenocorticotropic hormone. J Immunol 145:4326–4331

Brooks KH (1990) Adrenocorticotropin (ACTH) functions as a late-acting B-cell growth factor and synergizes with interleukin-5. J Mol Cell Immunol 4:327–337

Buzzetti R, Velente L, Barletta C, Scavo D, Possilli P (1989) Thymopentin induces release of ACTH-like immunoreactivity by human lymphocytes. J Clin Lab Immunol 29:157–159

Catania A, Airaghi L, Manfredi MG, Vivirito MC, Lipton JM (1992) Relations among plasma concentrations of alpha-MSH, ACTH and cytokines in AIDS patients. Endocrine Society 74th annual meeting, abstract no 591

Chang ACY, Cochet M, Cohen SN (1980) Structural organization of human genomic DNA encoding the pro-opiomelanocortin peptide. Proc Natl Acad Sci USA 77:4890–4894

Clarke BL, Bost KL (1989) Differential expression of functional adrenocorticotropic hormone receptors by subpopulations of lymphocytes. J Immunol 143:464–469

DiAugustine RP, Lazarus LH, Jahnke G, Khan MN, Erisman MD, Linnoila RI (1980) Corticotropin/beta-endorphin immunoreactivity in rat mast cells. Peptide or protease? Life Sci 27:2663–2666

Dupont AG, Somers G, Van Steirteghem AC, Warson F, Vanhelst L (1984) Ectopic adrenocorticotropin production: disappearance after removal of inflammatory tissue. J Clin Endocrinol Metab 58:654–658

Duvaux-Miret O, Capron A (1991) Pro-opiomelanocortin gene and gene products: a comparative study. Adv Neuroimmunol 1:41–57

Duvaux-Miret O, Stefano GB, Smith EM, Dissous C, Capron A (1992) Immunosuppression in the definitive and intermediate hosts of the human parasite *Schistosoma mansoni* by release of immunoactive neuropeptides. Proc Natl Acad Sci USA 89:778–781

Galin FS, LeBoeuf RD, Blalock JE (1990) A lymphocyte mRNA encodes the adrenocorticotropin/B-lipotropin region of the pro-opiomelanocortin gene. Prog Neuroendocrinimmunol 3:205–208

Hansen BL, Hansen GN, Scharrer B (1986) Immunocytochemical demonstration of a material resembling vertebrate ACTH and MSH in the corpus cardiacum–corpus allatum complex of the insect *Leucophaea maderae*. In: Stefano GB (ed) Handbook of comparative aspects of opioid and related neuropeptide mechanisms vol 1. CRC Press, Boca Raton, pp 213–222

Harbour DV, Smith EM, Blalock JE (1987) Novel pathway for proopiomelanocortin in lymphocytes: endotoxin induction of a new prohormone-cleaving enzyme. J Neurosci Res 18:95–101

Harbour-McMenamin DV, Smith EM, Blalock JE (1985) Bacterial lipopolysaccharide induction of leukocyte-derived corticotropin and endorphins. Infect Immun 48:813–817

Harper M, Marselle LM, Gallo RC, Wong-Staal F (1986) Detection of lymphocytes expressing human T-lymphotropic virus type III in lymph nodes and peripheral blood from infected individuals: in situ hybridization. Proc Natl Acad Sci USA 83:772–776

Hashemi FB, Hughes TK, Smith EM (1992) Characterization of immunoreactive corticotropin in lymphocytes infected with human immunodeficiency virus. American Society of Microbiology annual meeting, abstract

Heijnen CJ, Zulstra J, Kavelaars A, Croiset G, Ballieux RE (1987) Modulation of the immune response by POMC-derived peptides. Brain Behav Immun 1:284–291

Hirsch MD, O'Donohue TL (1986) Structural modifications of pro-opiomelanocortin-derived peptides alter their behavioral effects. J Pharmacol Exp Ther 237:378–395

Hughes TK, Smith EM (1990) Corticotropin (ACTH) induction of tumor necrosis factor-alpha by monocytes. J Biol Regul Homeost Agents 3:163–166

Johnson EW (1989) Distribution, modulation, and function of murine leukocyte adrenocorticotropin receptors. PhD dissertation. University of Texas Medical Branch, Galveston

Johnson EW, Blalock JE, Smith EM (1988) ACTH receptor induction of leukocyte cyclic AMP. Biochem Biophys Res Commun 157:1205–1211

Johnson HM, Smith EM, Torres BA, Blalock JE (1982) Regulation of the in vitro antibody response by neuroendocrine hormones. Proc Natl Acad Sci USA 79:4171–4174

Johnson HM, Torres BA, Smith EM, Dion LD, Blalock JE (1984) Regulation of lymphokine (gamma-interferon) production by corticotropin. J Immunol 132:246–250

Kavelaars A, Ballieux RE, Heijnen C (1988) Modulation of the immune response by pro-opiomelanocortin-derived peptides. Brain Behav Immun 2:57–66

Kavelaars A, Ballieux RE, Heijnen C (1989) The role of interleukin-1 in the corticotropin-releasing factor and arginine vasopressin-induced secretion of immunoreactive B-endorphin by human peripheral blood mononuclear cells. J Immunol 142:2338–2343

Koff WC, Dunegan MA (1985) Modulation of macrophage-mediated tumoricidal activity of neuropeptides and neurohormones. J Immunol 135:350–354

Krieger DT (1983) The multiple faces of pro-opiomelanocortin, a prototype precursor molecule. Clin Res 31:342–353

Krieger DT, Liotta A, Brownstein MJ (1977) Presence of adrenocorticotropin in brain of normal and hypophysectomized rats. Proc Natl Acad Sci USA 74:648–652

Lacaze-Masmonteil T, DeKeyzer Y, Luton J, Kahn P, Bertagnea X (1987) Characterization of proopiomelanocortin transcripts in human nonpituitary tissues. Proc Natl Acad Sci USA 84:7261–7264

Larsson L (1981) Adrenocorticotropin-like and alpha-melanotropin-like peptides in a subpopulation of human gastrin cell granules: bioassay, immunoassay, and immunocytochemical evidence. Proc Natl Acad Sci USA 78:1990–1993

Leach L, Trudaill DL, Gahan PB (1987) Immunocytochemical localization of neurosecretory amines and peptides in the free-living nematode, Goodeyus alm. Histochemical J 19:471–475

LeRoith E, Liotta AS, Roth J, Shiloach J, Lewis ME, Pert CB, Krieger DT (1982) ACTH and beta-endorphin-like materials are native to unicellular organisms. Proc Natl Acad Sci USA 79:2086–2090

Li CH (1972) Adrenocorticotropin 45. Revised amino acid sequences for sheep and bovine hormones. Biochem Biophys Res Commun 49:835–829

Liotta AS, Krieger DT (1983) Proopiomelanocortin (POMC) related peptides in rat brain differ in covalent modification from those in pars intermedia (PI) Proceedings of the 65th Endocrine Society meeting

Liotta AS, Osathanondh R, Krieger DT (1977) Presence of ACTH in human placenta:demonstration of in vitro synthesis. Endocrinology 101:1552–1558

Lolait SJ, Lim AJW, Toh BH, Funder JW (1984) Immunoreactive beta-endorphin in a subpopulation of mouse macrophages. J Clin Invest 73:277–280

Margioris A, Liotta AS, Vaudry H, Bardin CW, Krieger DT (1983) Characterization of immunoreactive proopiomelanocortin-related peptides in rat testes Endocrinology 113:663–671

McGillis JP, Park A, Rubin-Fletter P, Turck C, Dallman MF, Payan DG (1989) Stimulation of rat B-lymphocyte proliferation by corticotropin-releasing factor. J Neurosci Res 23:346–352

Munck A, Guyre PM, Holbrook NJ (1984) Physiological functions of glucocorticoids in stress and their relation to pharmacological actions. Endocrin Rev 5:25–44

Munn NA, Lum LG (1989) Immunoregulatory effects of alpha-endorphin, beta-endorphin, methionine-enkephalin, and adrenocorticotropic hormone on anti-tetanus toxoid antibody synthesis by human lymphocytes. Clin Immunol Immunopathol 52:376–385

Oates EL, Allaway GP, Armstrong GR, Boyajian RA, Kehrl JH, Prabhaker BS (1988) Human lymphocytes produce pro-opiomelanocortin gene-related transcripts. J Biol Chem 263:10041–10044

Oates EL, Allaway GP, Prabhakar BS (1990) A potential for mutual regulation of proopiomelanocortin gene and Epstein-Barr virus expression in human lymphocytes, Ann NY Acad Sci 594:60–65

O'Donohue TL, Holmquist GE, Jacobowitz DM (1979) Effect of hypophysectomy on alpha-melanotropin in discrete regions of the rat brain. Neurosci Lett 14:271–274

Ottaviani E, Petraglia F, Montagnani G, Cossarizza A, Monti D, Franceschi C (1990) Presence of ACTH and beta-endorphin immunoreactive molecules in the freshwater snail Planorbarius corneus (L.) (Gastropoda, Pulmonata) and their possible role in phagocytosis. Regul Pept 27:1–9

Ottaviani E, Caselgrandi E, Bondi M, Cossarizza A, Monti D, Franceschi C (1991) The "immune-mobile brain:"evolutionary evidence. Adv Neuroimmunol 1:27–39

Rafaeli A, Moshitzky P, Applebaum SW (1987) Diuretic action and immunological cross-reactivity of corticotropin and locust diuretic hormone. Gen Comp Endocrinol 67:1–6

Rivier J, Spiess J, Vale W (1983) Characterization of rat hypothalamic corticotropin-releasing factor. Proc Natl Acad Sci USA 80:4851–4855

Schols D, Verhaert P, Huybrechts R, Vaudry H, Jegou S, DeLoof A (1987) Immunocytochemical demonstration of proopiomelanocortin- and other opioid-related substances and a CRF-like peptide in the gut of the American cockroach. *Periplaneta americana L* Histochemistry 86:345–351

Shipp MA, Stefano GB, D'Adamio L, Switzer SN, Howard FD, Sinisterra J, Scharrer B, Reinherz EI (1990) Downregulation of enkephalin-mediated inflammatory responses by CD10/neutral endopeptidase 24.11. Nature 347:394–396

Singh (1989) Stimulatory effect of corticotropin–releasing neurohormone on human lymphocyte proliferation and interleukin-2 receptor expression. J Neuroimmunol 23:257–262

Smith AI, Funder JW (1988) Proopiomelanocortin processing in the pituitary, central nervous system, and peripheral tissues. Endocr Rev 9:159–179

Smith EM, Blalock JE (1981) Human leukocyte production of corticotropin and endorphin-like substances: association with leukocyte interferon. Proc Natl Acad Sci USA 78:7530–7534

Smith EM, Johnson EW (1988) A molecular basis for bi-directional communication between the neuroendocrine and immune systems. In: Hadden JW, Spreafico F, Yamamura Y. Austen KF, Dukor P, Masek K (eds) *Advances in immunopharmacology IV*. Pergamon Oxford, pp 47–54

Smith EM, Meyer WJ, Blalock JE (1982) Virus-induced corticosterone in hypophysectomized mice: a possible lymphoid-adrenal axis. Science 218:1311–1312

Smith EM, Morrill AC, Meyer WJ, Blalock JE (1986) Corticotropin releasing factor induction of leukocyte-derived immunoreactive ACTH and endorphins. Nature 321:881–882

Smith EM, Brosnan P, Meyer WJ, Blalock JE (1987) A corticotropin (ACTH) receptor on human mononuclear lymphocytes: correlation with adrenal ACTH receptor activity. N Engl J Med 317:1266–1269

Smith EM, Galin FS, LeBouf RD, Coppenhaver DH, Harbour DV, Blalock JE (1990a) Nucleotide and amino acid sequence of lymphocyte-derived corticotropin: endotoxin induction of a truncated peptide. Proc Natl Acad Sci USA 84:1057–1060

Smith EM, Hughes TK, Scharrer B, Leung MK, Stefano GB (1990b) the production and action of ACTH-related peptides in invertebrate hemocytes. 1st Int Con ISNIM, abstract no 39

Smith EM, Hughes TK, Hashemi F, Stefano GB (1992) Immunosuppressive effects of corticotropin and melanotropin and their possible significance in human immunodeficiency virus infection. Proc Natl Acad Sci USA 89:782–786

Stefano GB, Cadet P, Scharrer B (1989) Stimulatory effects of opioid neuropeptides on locomotory activity and conformational changes in invertebrate and human immunocytes: evidence for a subtype of δ-receptor. Proc Natl Acad Sci USA 86:6307–6311

Stefano GB, Smith DM, Smith EM, Hughes TK (1991) MSH can deactivate both TNF stimulated and spontaneously active immunocytes. In: Kits KS, Boer HH, Joosse J (eds) *Molluscan neurobiology*. North Holland, Amsterdam, pp 206–209

Strand FL, Rose KJ, Zuccarelli LA, Kume J, Alves SE, Antonawich FJ, Garrett LY (1991) Neuropeptide hormones as neurotrophic factors. Physiol Rev 71:1017–1046

Tanaka I, Nakai Y, Nakao K, Oki S, Masaki N, Ohtsuki H, Imura H (1982) Presence of immunoreactive-alpha melanocyte stimulating hormone, adrenocorticotropin, and beta-endorphin in human gastric antral mucosa. J Clin Endocrinol Metab 54:392–396

Van Epps DE, Mason MM (1990) Modulation of leukocyte migration by alpha-melanocyte stimulating hormone. In: Stefano GB, Florey E (eds) *Comparative pharmacology of neuropeptides*. Manchester University Press, Manchester, pp 335–345

Verges B, Chavanet P, Desgres J, Vaillant G, Waldner A, Brun JM, Putelat R (1989) Adrenal function in HIV infected patients. Acta Endocrinol (Copenh) 121:633–637

Ways DK, Zimmerman CF, Ontjes DA (1976) Inhibition of adrenocorticotropin effects on adrenal cell membranes by synthetic adrenocorticotropin analogues: correlation of binding and adenylate cyclase activation. Mol Pharmacol 12:789–799

Webster EL, Battaglia G, DeSouza EB (1989) Functional corticotropin-releasing factor (CRF) receptors in mouse spleen: evidence from adenylate cyclase studies. Peptides 10:395–401

Webster EL, DeSouza EB (1988) Corticotropin-releasing receptors in mouse spleen: identification, autoradiographic localization, and regulation by divalent and guanine nucleotides. Endocrinology 122:609–617

Westly HJ, Kleiss AJ, Kelley KW, Wong PKY, Yuen P (1986) Newcastle disease virus-infected splenocytes express the pro-opiomelanocortin gene. J Exp Med 163:1589–1594

α-Melanotropin and its Role in Regulating the Inflammatory Response

D. E. Van Epps

Introduction

Melanotropins (MSH) are widely distributed in vertebrates and invertebrates. Originally defined by their effect on amphibian melanocytes—darkening their skin as a defense mechanism—these peptides have additional functions that are as yet less well understood. There are three melanocyte stimulating hormones, α-, β-, and γ-MSH, derived from a 31-kDa precursor in the pituitary gland. Of particular interest to the immunologist are α-MSH and γ-MSH. γ-MSH has been found in neutrophils as measured by reactivity with specific anti-γ-MSH antibody (Vaalasti and Johansson 1988). α-MSH, on the other hand, has recently been shown to modulate cytokine-induced inflammatory reactions, fever, and acute-phase reactant release in vivo (reviewed in Lipton 1988). In addition, α-MSH stimulates nerve regeneration (Bijlsma et al. 1983). These observations bring new light to the possible functions of MSH, extending them beyond a highly specific action on melanocytes. This chapter focuses on the role of α-MSH in regulating the inflammatory process and the associated physiological response.

Nature of α-MSH

α-MSH is a 13 amino acid peptide which is homologous to the first 13 amino acids of adrenocorticotropic hormone (ACTH) and by inference is a component of pro-opiomelanocortin (POMC). It was first isolated from porcine pituitary glands by Lerner and Lee (1955), and its structure was determined in 1957 (Harris and Lerner 1957). Figure 1 shows the cleavage peptides derived from the 31-kDa POMC precursor protein molecule in the intermediate lobe of the pituitary and the amino acid sequences of the three forms of MSH present in POMC. α-MSH and several other immunomodulating peptides including ACTH, β-endorphin,

Applied Science Immunotherapy Division, Baxter Healthcare Corp., Round Lake, IL, USA

Scharrer et al. (Eds.)
Neuropeptides and Immunoregulation

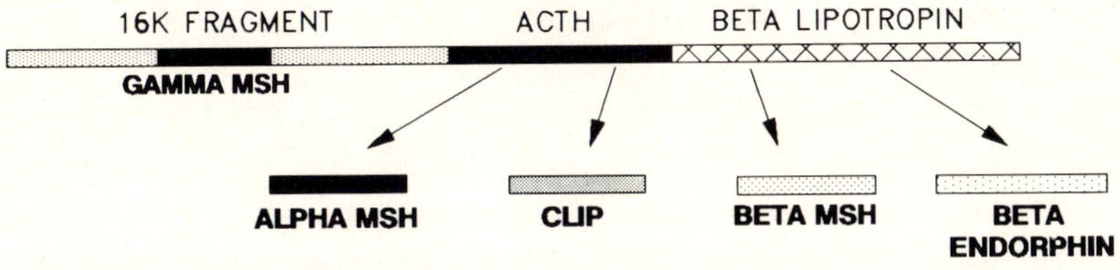

AMINO ACID SEQUENCE OF DIFFERENT MSH SPECIES

ALPHA MSH	**SER-TYR-SER-MET-GLU-HIS-PHE-ARG-TRP-GLY-LYS-PRO-VAL**
BETA MSH	**ALA-GLU-LYS-LYS-ASP-GLU-GLY-PRO-TYR-ARG-MET-GLU-HIS-PHE-ARG-TRP-GLY-SER-PRO-PRO-LYS-ASP**
GAMMA MSH	**TYR-VAL-MET-GLY-HIS-PHE-ARG-TRP-ASP-ARG-PHE-GLY**

Fig. 1. Sources of MSH from POMC and comparative amino acid sequences of α-, β-, and γ-MSH

and Met-enkephalin are all derived from POMC through differential processing of the precursor peptide by the action of specific enzymes. In addition to its presence in the intermediate lobe of the pituitary, α-MSH occurs in MSH-containing neurons in the hypothalamus, thalamus, midbrain, amygdala, septum, and cortex (Shizame 1985). α-MSH has also been identified in mucosal and muscular layers of the gastrointestinal tract (Fox and Kricer 1981) and in the peripheral circulation (Kortlandt et al. 1986).

As with several pituitary neuropeptides, α-MSH levels are elevated under conditions of stress, including immobilization (Khorram et al. 1985) and transient exposure of rats to ether (Usategui et al. 1976). Other studies have shown that α-MSH is increased in the peripheral circulation during the third trimester of pregnancy (Clark et al. 1978). These observations suggest that α-MSH acts systemically in response to stress and makes it a good candidate for immunoregulation, as is the case with other neuroendocrine peptides such as ACTH, β-endorphin, Met-enkephalin, and vasoactive intestinal peptide (see Weigent and Blalock, this volume). Much like ACTH, α-MSH has also been shown to be increased in the plasma of rats following treatment with corticotropin-releasing factor (CRF), again indicating a peripheral action of α-MSH in response to stress or to the presence of CRF (Proulx-Ferland et al. 1983). Further evidence that α-MSH acts systemically and may have a broad spectrum of activities comes from studies in rodents, indicating that specific receptors for α-MSH are widely distributed in glandular organs such as the adrenals, pancreas, and lacrimal glands as well as in the adipose tissues, bladder, duodenum, skin, spleen, and hypothalamus (Tatro and Reichlin 1987). This widespread expression of α-MSH receptors on a variety of cell types implies important biological functions for α-MSH.

Antipyretic Effects of α-MSH

α-MSH, as well as its precursor molecule ACTH, has been shown to have antipyretic activity and to reduce fever induced by the injection of endotoxin (Glyn and Lipton 1982). High concentrations of α-MSH and ACTH can reduce body temperature in afebrile animals. Lower concentrations which do not cause temperature reduction in afebrile animals are still able to prevent fever in response to pyretic agents (Lipton 1988). Although α-MSH was initially shown to reduce the pyrogenic response to endotoxin, it also is effective at inhibiting hyperthermia in response to natural and recombinant interleukin-1 (IL-1), which is one of the presumed mediators of the pyrogenic reaction (reviewed in Lipton 1988). Its antipyretic activity has been shown in rabbits (Lipton 1988), guinea pigs (Kandasamy and Williams 1984), squirrel monkeys (Shih and Lipton 1985), and mice (Robertson et al. 1986).

α-MSH has been shown to have antipyretic activity when injected directly into the central nervous system (CNS) at a dose as low as 25 ng (Murphy et al. 1983). In comparative studies 200 ng α-MSH was equivalent to 500 μg acetaminophen in reduction of the fever response to intravenous injection of endogenous pyrogen (IL-1). These data suggest that by this route of administration α-MSH is 2500 times more potent in its antipyretic effect than acetaminophen. Interestingly, although α-MSH has potent antipyretic activity when used in conjunction with endotoxin or IL-1, it has little effect on the fever induced by arachidonate or prostaglandin E_2 (PGE_2; Clark et al. 1985). This differs from the observations with acetaminophen, which inhibits arachidonate-induced fever but not PGE_2-induced fever, suggesting that the antipyretic effect of α-MSH differs in its mechanism of action compared to acetaminophen, which acts directly on arachidonate metabolism pathways.

Data suggesting that α-MSH may act as a CNS regulator of the febrile response come from studies by Samson et al. (1981) showing that in rabbits the injection of IL-1 and the consequent febrile response are associated with an increase in α-MSH in the septal region of the brain. This observation was confirmed by a study by Holdeman et al. (1985) in which septum MSH was increased with IL-1 injection, but not by heat exposure to induce hyperthermia. These two studies, along with the evidence that systemic injection of α-MSH can also inhibit the fever reaction to pyrogens, indicate that α-MSH may serve a central role in thermal regulation.

More evidence supporting the antipyretic action of α-MSH comes from studies by Shih et al. (1986) in which a specific rabbit anti-α-MSH antiserum was injected intraventricularly, followed by an intravenous injection of IL-1. Under these conditions the fever induced by IL-1 was greatly prolonged in animals receiving anti-α-MSH treatment, suggesting that the blocking of α-MSH activity prevents the natural regulation of fever.

Additional evidence indicating that α-MSH is involved in the regulation of pyrogen-induced fever comes from studies of Sawyer et al. (1984) with an α-MSH analog differing in positions 7 and 4 (Fig. 1) where D-phenylalanine and norleucine are substituted for methionine and phenylalanine, respectively. This analog has a prolonged half-life compared to α-MSH and is resistant to enzymatic digestion. It was found to be much more potent than α-MSH in the reduction of fever induced by IL-1 when injected intracranially but had little activity when injected systemically, suggesting either an alteration of the peptide in the peripheral circulation or a failure of the peptide to cross the blood-brain barrier.

The active region of the α-MSH peptide has been studied by Lipton (1988), who found that neither the 1–10 nor the 4–10 amino acid peptides of α-MSH have antipyretic activity. It was subsequently found that the tripeptide 11–13, Lys-Pro-Val, is able to reduce fever when given centrally or peripherally, although its potency is somewhat less than that of α-MSH itself (Richards and Lipton 1984). These data suggest that the three carboxyl terminal amino acids are actively involved in the antipyretic activity of α-MSH.

Role of α-MSH in the Modulation of the IL-1 Mediated Response

Although IL-1 is known to be pyrogenic, its function goes well beyond the induction of fever and includes stimulation of the release of ACTH from the pituitary (Dinarello and Wolff 1982) and of serum amyloid protein (SAP) from hepatocytes (Robertson et al. 1986), induction of leukocytosis, triggering prostaglandin production by synovial cells (Dayer et al. 1986) and fibroblasts (Cannon et al. 1986), stimulation of increased adhesiveness of neutrophils (PMN) to endothelial cells (Bevilacqua et al. 1985; Dunn and Fleming 1985; Gamble et al. 1985; Pohlman et al. 1986; Schleimer and Rutledge 1986), and mediation of the mobilization of PMN to inflammatory sites in vivo (reviewed in Van Epps 1991). All of these steps are critical to mounting a normal inflammatory response to an invading organism or an antigen. In addition to IL-1, many other endogenous peptides can stimulate an inflammatory reaction, such as the cytokines tumor necrosis factor-α (TNF-α) and IL-8 or neutrophil-activating peptide (NAP-1). This inflammatory response is brought about directly or indirectly. In addition, peptides such as C5a derived from the complement system can trigger an inflammatory response along with the associated influx of neutrophils (Mason and Van Epps 1989a).

The role of α-MSH as an antipyretic following injection of IL-1 is not limited to this in vivo response. Most studies indicate that α-MSH has a broad effect on the acute-phase reaction stimulated by IL-1. This reaction includes fever, leukocytosis, and the elevation of serum reactive protein, SAP, and plasma corticosterone levels, to name a few. In this regard, Robertson et al. (1986) showed in mice that 30 μg α-MSH administered peripherally is able to suppress the IL-1-induced fever, neutropenia, and SAP responses. This inhibition was dose dependent and could be overcome by the injection of excess IL-1. In these studies neither ACTH nor glucocorticoids could duplicate the inhibitory activity observed with α-MSH. In addition, these investigators found that if α-MSH is administered 1–2 h prior to IL-1, no effect on the IL-1 responses is observed, suggesting a limited lifespan for the α-MSH mediated activity. This may be related to the very short half-life of α-MSH in vivo (2.5 min; Kastin et al. 1976).

Interestingly, in in vitro assays which measure the capacity of IL-1 to costimulate mitogenic responses of murine thymocytes, α-MSH had no effect, indicating that α-MSH does not act through a direct inhibition of the IL-1 receptor on these cells. This is further supported by other in vitro studies (Daynes et al. 1987) which show that both the IL-1-induced increases in plasma glucocorticoids and the ability of IL-1 to inhibit contact hypersensitivity are blocked by α-MSH while IL-1 induced PGE elevation in plasma is not. Additional in vitro studies showed that α-MSH fails to inhibit IL-1 stimulated production of PGE by fibroblasts and IL-1 induced thymocyte proliferation. The lack of an effect of α-MSH on IL-1 induced PGE production was also confirmed in a system in which rat astrocytes were used as the target cells (Katsuura et al. 1989). In contrast to these studies, however, Cannon et al. (1986) have shown that α-MSH inhibits IL-1 induced PGE production by fibroblasts and thymocyte proliferation in response to IL-1. In their studies the inhibitory activity was observed with low concentrations (10^{-11}–10^{-8} *M*) while higher concentrations showed less activity. In addition, the potent α-MSH analog Nle^4, *d*-Phe^7 MSH did not have any effect on the IL-1 induced thymocyte proliferation. It is not clear at this time what accounts for the differences among the studies by Robertson et al. (1986), Daynes et al. (1987), Katsuura et al. (1989), and Cannon et al. (1986).

Role of α-MSH in Modulating the Inflammatory Reaction

Studies by Lipton (1988) in rabbits have shown that the terminal tripeptide of α-MSH, Ac-Lys-Pro-Val, is able to suppress histamine-induced edema in the skin when the peptide is injected intravenously 30 min prior to histamine. These data suggest that the action of this α-MSH peptide extends beyond suppression of IL-1 mediated fever and acute-phase release of the reactant. Still other studies by Hiltz and Lipton (1989) have shown that in mice the injection of this tripeptide reduced the ear swelling response to picryl chloride as measured 3 and 6 h following exposure. As with the studies of histamine-induced edema, it is apparent that the α-MSH peptide has multiple activities, acting both as an antipyretic and a general suppressor of inflammatory reactions. If these data with tripeptide can be extrapolated to α-MSH, it may be that this neuropeptide functions as a natural regulator of inflammation.

Studies supporting the hypothesis that α-MSH is a natural regulator of the inflammatory process have been performed using a murine model of the inflammatory response mediated by IL-1, TNF-α and C5a (Mason and Van Epps

1989b). In these studies, 1-cm^2 collagen sponges were implanted subcutaneously in the flank and shoulder regions of C3H/ouj mice. After a 48-h recovery period sponges were injected through the skin with 0.1 ml TNF-α, IL-1-β, or purified human C5a. At varying times after the injection sponges were removed and subjected to collagenase; the cell suspension obtained was counted and stained for microscopic analysis. This model system can be used to quantitate the number and types of cells migrating into the sponges in response to a known inflammatory stimulus (Mason and Van Epps 1989). In this model, the maximal cellular infiltrate occurred 6 h after the injection of sponges. The response to IL-1, C5a, or TNF-α was predominantly an increase in PMN. The most abundant cell type in the sponge was the macrophage. However, there was relatively little change in the absolute number of these cells or of lymphocytes in TNF-α-, IL-1-, or C5a-injected sponges compared to control sponges at any time over a 24-h period.

Using this model system it was possible to determine whether intraperitoneal injection of α-MSH is able to modulate the mobilization of neutrophils in response to specific inflammatory stimuli. When mice were injected intraperitoneally with

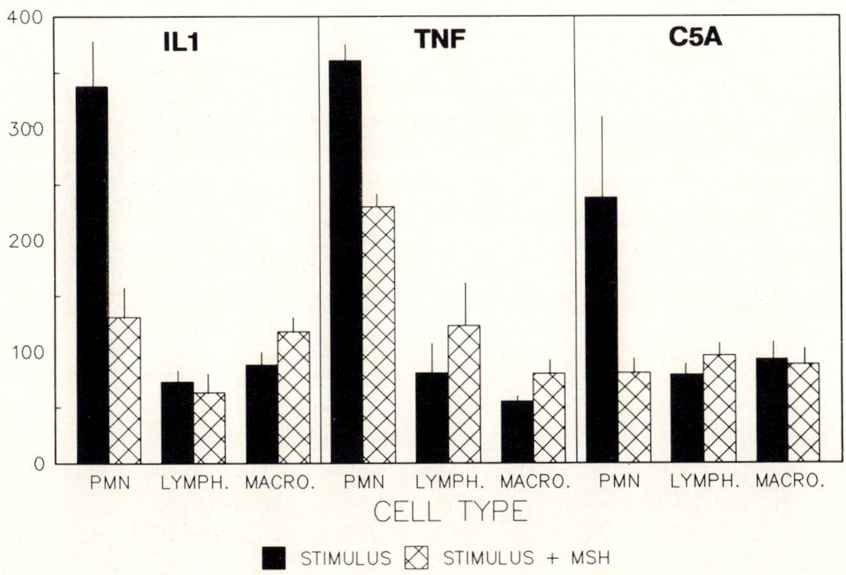

Fig. 2. Effect of α-MSH on the migration of PMN, monocytes, and lymphocytes into subcutaneous collagen-sponge implants 6 h after injection of 5 U IL-1, 0.2 μg TNF-α, or 0.1 ml 10^{-7} *M* C5a. In each case 0.1 ml 10^{-5} *M* α-MSH was injected intraperitoneally simultaneously with the stimulatory agent into the sponge. The data show the mean ±SD for at least six collagen sponges in each case. *Solid bars*, response to the indicated stimulus without injection of α-MSH; *hatched bars*, response with simultaneous α-MSH injection. All data presented as percentage of the number of cells migrating into uninjected control cells, which ranged from approximately $1–3 \times 10^5$ for PMN, $1–3 \times 10^5$ for lymphocytes, and $9–14 \times 10^5$ for marcrophages. All results represent the response of cells 6 h after injection of stimulatory agent into implants

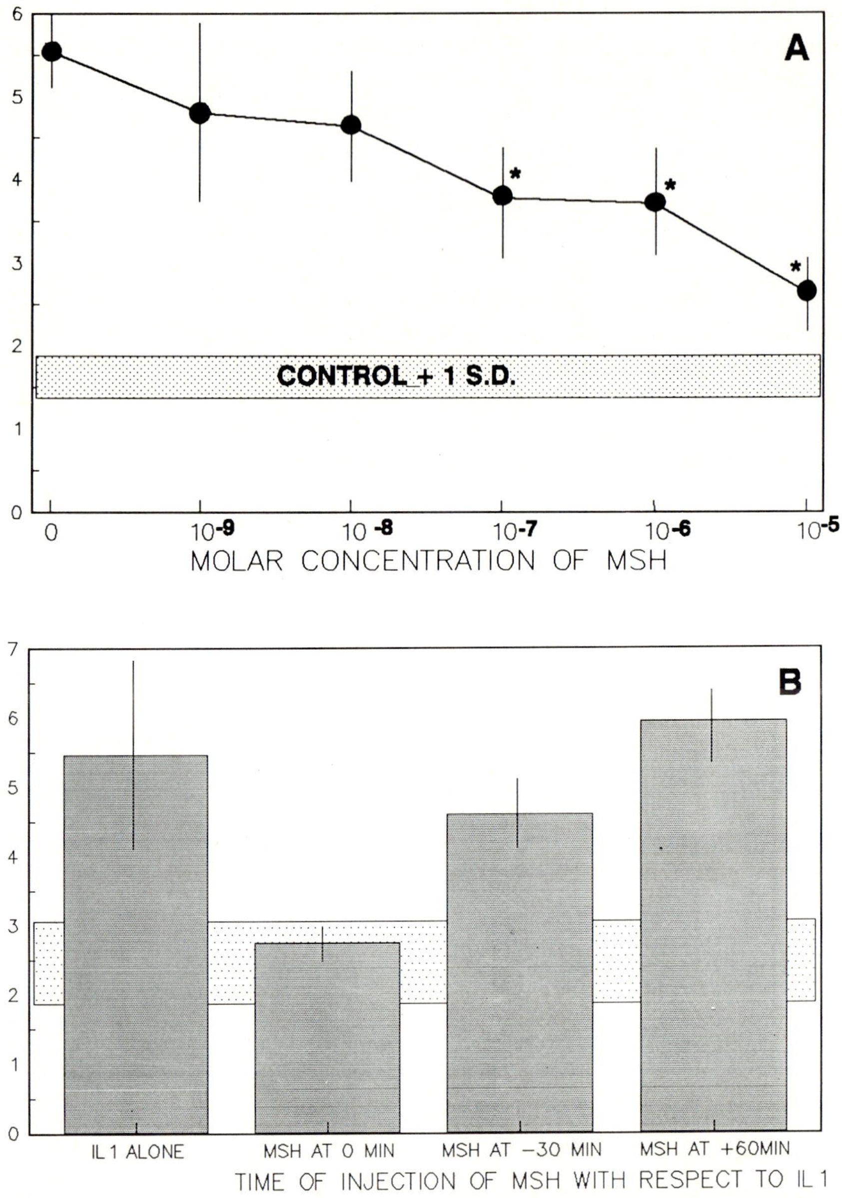

Fig. 3. A Dose-response curve for α-MSH inhibition of PMN migration into collagen sponges in vivo in response to 5 U IL-1. Each point represents the mean response for a minimum of six sponges; standard deviations indicated at each point. All responses measured at 6 h after intraperitoneal injection of 10^{-5} *M* α-MSH and sponge injection of IL-1. *Stippled area*, mean ± 1 SD for control responses in 12 different sponges. **B** Time dependence for α-MSH inhibition of IL-1 mediated emigration of PMN into collagen sponges in the mouse. *Bars*, mean PMN response to IL-1 ± 1 SD with or without intraperitoneal injection of 5 U IL-1 and 10^{-5} *M* α-MSH simultaneously, 30 min. *Stippled area*, mean ± 1 SD for saline-injected control sponges

0.1 ml 10^{-5} *M* α-MSH simultaneously with the injection of 0.2 μg TNF-α, 5 U IL-1, or 10^{-7} *M* C5a, a marked reduction in the mobilization of PMN into the implants at 6 h was observed (Fig. 2). This reduction in response applied only to PMN; there were no major differences in the numbers of lymphocytes or monocytes/macrophages present in sponges injected with stimulatory substances compared to control sponges. Additional dose-response studies showed that the effect of α-MSH on the immigration of PMN was dose dependent, with a significant decrease first observed after the injection of as little as 10^{-8} *M* α-MSH (Fig. 3A).

These studies support the hypothesis that α-MSH is a general regulator of the inflammatory process, and that its activity extends beyond its mere antipyretic activity. Furthermore, it is clear from these studies that α-MSH can act systemically to inhibit PMN migration since the site of injection of α-MSH was intraperitoneal, whereas the site of injection of inflammatory agents was intradermal. Finally, these studies indicate that the mode of action of α-MSH in modulating the inflammatory reaction is not due to a specific inhibition of IL-1 receptors since its effect was observed with multiple stimuli including TNF-α and C5a. On the contrary, it can be assumed that the action of α-MSH in this system must involve some more basic and common component of the inflammatory process.

Additional studies performed to determine the temporal relationship of α-MSH injection and inhibition of the immigration of PMN in response to an inflammatory stimulus have shown that α-MSH is effective only when injected simultaneously with the injection of the inflammatory material since suppression of the PMN response to IL-1 was not observed when α-MSH was administered 30 min before or 1 h after the injection of the stimulatory substance (Fig. 3B; Mason and Van Epps 1989). This is similar to the results obtained by Robertson et al. (1986) in evaluating the action of α-MSH on acute-phase reactant release. There is also an apparent structural specificity of α-MSH regarding its inhibitory effect since ACTH, which contains the α-MSH sequence, showed much less activity than α-MSH (Mason and Van Epps 1989b). These data are also comparable to those obtained in vivo with IL-1 mediated acute-phase reactant release when ACTH had little effect (Daynes et al. 1987).

Although it is still unclear how α-MSH functions as an immunoregulator, or what mechanism is involved, this peptide can be considered a potent general suppressor of host responses to inflammatory stimuli. Its activity ranges from that of an antipyretic to that of an inhibitor of PMN mobilization to an inflammatory site. The antipyretic activity, along with studies by Lipton (1988) and coworkers showing an effective action of CNS-injected α-MSH, suggests that the action of α-MSH may be due at least in part to an action of the CNS. The concept that α-MSH may alter the inflammatory response to a variety of stimuli via this indirect pathway is supported by the large body of information on the link between the CNS and the immune system. It is also possible that by lowering vascular permeability α-MSH may reduce the movement of mobilized PMN to an inflammatory site (Mason and Van Epps 1989b), reduce histamine induced edema (Lipton 1988), and suppress the ear swelling reaction to picryl chloride (Hiltz and Lipton 1989). Which of these possibilities is in fact the case remains to be determined. However, it is clear that α-MSH does not act solely through inhibition of IL-1 binding to its receptor, as speculated by some investigators (Cannon et al. 1986), since it appears to act only on in vivo IL-1 mediated responses and not on in vitro responses. Furthermore, its broad activity and specificity is characteristic of a more generalized mechanism.

Recent studies by Rheins et al. (1989) have shown that epicutaneous application of α-MSH suppresses contact hypersensitivity to both dinitrofluorobenzene and oxazalone in mice. This loss of contact hypersensitivity could be reversed by intradermal or intravenous injection of IL-1, a result that again suggests a regulatory role for α-MSH in the inflammatory reaction.

The release of α-MSH under conditions of stress supports the concept that α-MSH may be a true immunoregulator much like glucocorticoids or opioid peptides. Its very short half-life and the necessity that it be administered simultaneously with the inflammatory stimulus also support such a role. It may be speculated that ACTH released in response to IL-1 into the circulation could act as the precursor molecule for α-MSH. Local cleavage of ACTH could yield α-MSH, suppressing the events mediated by IL-1 or other cytokines (see also Smith, this volume). It is well known that IL-1 can stimulate ACTH release from the pituitary (Besedovsky et al. 1986) and in some cases from mononuclear leukocytes (Smith et al. 1986; Westly et al. 1986) although the latter may be somewhat controversial (Sobel 1990). A sequence of active IL-1 production, release of α-MSH and/or its precursor molecule ACTH, suppression of the pyretic response, acute-phase reaction, and the inflammatory response would seem to be a suitable mechanism to control an overactivated inflammatory reaction.

The hypothesis that MSH is a major natural regulator of cytokine-induced inflammation requires further proof. However, it is clear that the known functions of MSH in mammals can now be expanded to include a role for this peptide in thermal regulation in response to pyrogens and modulation of cytokine-mediated events.

References

Besedovsky H, DelRey A, Sorkin E, Dinarello CA (1986) Immunoregulatory feedback between interleukin-1 and glucocorticoid hormones. Science 233:652

Bevilacqua MP, Pober JS, Wheeler ME, Cotran RS, Gimbrone MA (1985) Interleukin-1 acts on cultured human vascular endothelium to increase the adherence of polymorphonuclear leukocytes, monocytes and related leukocyte cell lines. J Clin Invest 76:2003

Bijlsma WA, Schotman P, Jennekens FG, Gispen WH, DeWied D (1983) The enhanced recovery of sensorimotor function in rats is related to the melanotropic moiety of ACTH/MSH neuropeptides. Eur J Pharmacol 92:231–236

Cannon JG, Tatro JB, Reichlin S, Dinarello CA (1986) Alpha-melanocyte stimulating hormone inhibits immunostimulatory and inflammatory actions of interleukin-1. J Immunol 137: 2232–2236

Clark D, Thody AJ, Shuster S, Bowers II (1978) Immunoreactive alpha-MSH in human plasma in pregnancy. Nature 273:163–164

Clark WG, Holdeman M, Lipton JM (1985) Analysis of the antipyretic action of alpha-melanocyte stimulating hormone in rabbits. J Physiol (Lond) 359:459–465

Dayer JM, deRochemonteix B, Burrus B, Demczuk S, Dinarello CA (1986) Human recombinant IL-1 stimulates collagenase and prostaglandin E production by human synovial cells. J Clin Invest 77:645

Daynes RA, Robertson BA, Cho BH, Burnham DK, Newton R (1987) Alpha-melanocyte stimulating hormone exhibits target cell selectivity in its capacity to affect interleukin 1-inducible responses in vivo and in vitro. J Immunol 139:103–109

Dinarello CA, Wolff SM (1982) Molecular basis of fever in humans. Am J Med 72:799–819

Dunn CJ, Fleming WE (1985) The role of interleukin-1 in the inflammatory response with particular reference to endothelial cell-leukocyte adhesion. Prog Leuk Biol 2:45

Fox JA, Kricer J (1981) Immunoreactive alpha-melanocyte stimulating hormone, its distribution in the gastrointestinal tract of intact and hypophysectomized rats. Life Sci 28:2127–2132

Gamble JR, Harlan JM, Klebanhoff JS, Vadas MA (1985) Stimulation of the adherence of neutrophils to umbilical vein endothelium by human recombinant tumor necrosis factor. Proc Natl Acad Sci USA 82:8667

Glyn JR, Lipton JM (1982) Hypothermic and antipyretic effects of centrally administered ACTH (1–24) and alpha-melanotropin. Peptides 2:177–187

Harris JI, Lerner AB (1957) Amino-acid sequence of alpha-melanocyte stimulating hormone. Nature 179:1346–1347

Hiltz ME, Lipton JM (1989) Antiinflammatory activity of a COOH-terminal fragment of the neuropeptide alpha-MSH. FASEB 3:2282–2284

Holdeman M, Khorram O, Samson WK, Lipton JM (1985) Fever-specific changes in MSH and CRF concentrations. Am J Physiol 248:R125

Kandasamy SB, Williams BA (1984) Hypothermic and anti-pyretic effects of ACTH (1–24) and alpha-melanotropin in guinea pigs. Neuropharmacology 23:49

Kastin AJ, Nissen C, Nikolics K, Medzihradszky K, Coy DH, Teplan I, Schally AV (1976) Distribution of [^{3}H]-MSH in rat brain. Brain Res Bull 1:19–26

Katsuura G, Gottschall PE, Dahl RR, Arimura A (1989) Interleukin-1 beta increases prostaglandin E_2 in rat astrocyte cultures: modulatory effect of neuropeptides. Endocrinology 124:3125–3127

Khorram O, Bedran de Castro JC, McCann SM (1985) Stress-induced secretion of alpha-melanocyte stimulating hormone and its physiological role in modulating the secretion of prolactin and luteinizing hormone in the female rat. Endocrinology 117:2483–2489

Kortlandt W, DeRotte AA, Arts CJM, Croughs RJM, Thijssen JHH (1986) Characterization of alpha-MSH-like immunoreactivity in human plasma. Acta Endocrinol (Copenh) 113:175–180

Lerner AB, Lee TH (1955) Isolation of homogeneous melanocyte stimulating hormone from hog pituitary gland. J Am Chem Soc 77:1066–1067

Lipton JM (1988) MSH in CNS control of fever and its influence on inflammation/immune responses. In: Hadley ME (ed) The melanotropic peptides. CRC Press, Boca Raton, pp 97–113

Mason MJ, Van Epps DE (1989a) In vivo neutrophil emigration in response to interleukin-1 and tumor necrosis factor-alpha. J Leukoc Biol 45:62–68

Mason MJ, Van Epps DE (1989b) Modulation of IL-1, tumor necrosis factor, and C5a-mediated murine neutrophil migration by alpha-melanocyte stimulating hormone. J Immunol 142: 1646–1651

Murphy MT, Richards DB, Lipton JM (1983) Antipyretic potency of centrally administered alpha-melanocyte stimulating hormone. Science 221:192–193

Pohlman TH, Stanness KA, Beatty PG, Ochs HD, Harlan JM (1986) An endothelial cell surface factor(s) induced in vitro by lipopolysaccharide, interleukin-1, and tumor necrosis factor-alpha increases neutrophil adherence by a CD w/18-dependent mechanism. J Immunol 136:4548

Proulx-Ferland L, Meunier H, Cote J, Dumont D, Gagne B, Labrie F (1983) Multiple factors involved in the control of ACTH and alpha-MSH secretion. J Steroid Biochem 19:439–445

Rheins LA, Cotleur AL, Kleier RS, Hoppenjans WB, Saunder DN, Nordlund JJ (1989) Alpha-melanocyte stimulating hormone modulates contact hypersensitivity responsiveness in C57/BL6 mice. J Invest Dermatol 93:511–517

Richards DB, Lipton JM (1984) Effect of alpha-MSH 11–13 (lysine-proline-valine) on fever in the rabbit. Peptides 5:815

Robertson BA, Gahring LC, Daynes RA (1986) Neuropeptide regulation of interleukin-1 activities; capacity of alpha-melanocyte stimulating hormone to inhibit interleukin-1 inducible responses in vivo and in vitro exhibits target cell selectivity. Inflammation 10:371–385

Samson WK, Lipton JM, Zimmer JA, Glyn JR (1981) Effect of fever on central alpha-MSH concentrations in the rabbit. Peptides 2:419

Sawyer TK, Sanfilippo PJ, Hruby VJ, Engel MH, Heward CB, Burnett JB, Hadley ME (1984) 4-Norleucine-7-d-phenylalanine-alpha-melanocyte stimulating hormone: a highly potent alpha-melanotropin with ultralong biological activity. Proc Natl Acad Sci USA 77:5754

Schleimer RP, Rutledge BK (1986) Cultured human vascular endothelial cells acquire adhesiveness for neutrophils after stimulation with interleukin-1, endotoxin, and tumor-promoting phorbol diesters. J Immunol 136:649

Shih ST, Lipton JM (1985) Intravenous alpha-MSH reduces fever in squirrel monkeys. Peptides 6:685

Shih ST, Khorram O, Lipton JM, McCann SM (1986) Central administration of alpha-MSH antiserum augments fever in the rabbit. Am J Physiol 250:R803–R806

Shizame K (1985) Thirty-five years of progress in the study of MSH. Yale J Biol Med 58:561–570

Smith RM, Morrill AC, Meyer III WJ, Blalock JE (1986) Corticotropin releasing factor induction of leukocyte-derived immunoreactive ACTH and endorphins. Nature 321:881–882

Sobel DO (1990) Corticotropin releasing hormone and arginine vasopressin stimulation of ACTH and substance P in human mononuclear leukocytes. Endocr Res 16(2):283–292

Tatro JB, Reichlin S (1987) Specific receptors for alpha-melanocyte stimulating hormone are widely distributed in tissues of rodents. Endocrinology 121(5):1900–1907

Usategui R, Oliver C, Vaudry H, Lombardi G, Rozenberg I, Mourre AM (1976) Immunoreactive alpha-MSH and ACTH levels in rat plasma and pituitary. Endocrinology 98:189–196

Vaalasti A, Johansson O (1988) Immunocytochemical demonstration of gamma-melanocyte stimulating hormone-like immunoreactivity in human neutrophilic granulocytes. Blood 71:804–806

Van Epps DE (1991) Cytokine stimulated emigration of granulocytes in vivo. In: Coffey RG (ed) Granulocyte responses to cytokines: basic and clinical research. Dekker, New York, pp 351–372

Westly HJ, Kleiss AJ, Kelley KW, Wong PKY, Yuen PH (1986) Newcastle disease virus-infected splenocytes express the proopiomelanocortin gene. J Exp Med 163:1589–1594

Immunoregulation by Neuropeptides Other than Corticotropin and Melanotropin

D. V. Harbour[1]

Introduction

This chapter reviews current information on the participation of neuropeptides other than the pro-opiomelanocortin peptides in immunoregulatory processes. These activities include the transmission of signals via the neuroendocrine system to the immune system and of other, directly or indirectly acting signals addressed by various neuropeptides to the immune system. Thyrotropin-releasing hormone (TRH) and the other mediators of the hypothalamic-pituitary-thyroid (HPT) axis, i.e., thyrotropin (TSH), prolactin, and the thyroid hormones triiodothyronine and thyroxine, are discussed in some detail. In addition, the effects of certain hypophysiotropins other than TRH, of the hypothalamic nonapeptides vasopressin and oxytocin, and of several extrahypothalamic neuropeptides are reviewed.

Thyrotropin-Releasing Hormone

TRH is a very small neuropeptide which, according to Jackson and Reichlin (1974; Reichlin 1986a), has survived evolutionary scrutiny to be used as a regulator of pituitary TSH control. In this capacity TRH, being produced and released by hypothalamic neurons, is partially regulated by external stimuli. One important factor activating these neurons and thus the HPT axis is stress (for review see Ingbar and Braverman 1986). TRH neurons are located in regions heavily innervated by adrenergic and noradrenergic neurons, which are also involved in the stress response (Jackson and Reichlin 1974; Reichlin 1986a). Again, these molecules are produced by neurons whose production is influenced by external stimuli (stresses) to the CNS.

[1] Department of Human Biological Chemistry and Genetics and Microbiology, University of Texas Medical Branch, Galveston, TX 77550, USA

Scharrer et al. (Eds.)
Neuropeptides and Immunoregulation

Indirect Modulation of the Immune Response via the HPT Axis

A malfunction of the hypothalamic neurons providing TRH affects the activity of thyrotropin and the thyroid hormones and alters the regulation of other peptide hormones, prolactin, and growth hormones (discussed below). Since these hormones have immunomodulatory activities, TRH indirectly participates in the neuroendocrine control of immune processes. These include inflammatory or nonspecific defense responses as well as specific immune responses (discussed below).

During a stress response, TRH via its indirect effect on thyroid hormone function alters the metabolic rate. Under certain conditions, the downregulation of TRH by thyroid hormones may lead to T-cell impairment, thus indirectly altering an inflammatory or nonspecific immune response as well as a specific immune response. Another indirect influence of TRH on immune processes via thyroid hormones may be the partial reconstitution of an atrophied thymus (Pierpaoli and Sorkin 1972).

TSH regulated by TRH, as well as by somatostatin, has potent immunomodulatory effects including the enhancement of antibody response through a poorly characterized mechanism (Kruger and Blalock 1986; Kruger et al. 1990). Others have reported that TSH has an effect on natural killer (NK) cell function through the alteration of the IL-2 receptor expression and a decrease in iodine uptake and phagocytosis in phagocytic cells (Stolc 1972a, b; Chabaud and Lissitsky 1977; Provinciali and Fabris 1990). Lymphoid cells produce mature TSH protein and TSH mRNA in response to TRH (Harbour et al. 1988, 1989; Kruger et al. 1990). In addition to positive regulation by TRH, the immunoreactive (ir) TSH produced by Molt 4 T-cells is downregulated by triiodothyronine both at the level of the protein and the level of mRNA (Harbour et al. 1989), which ultimately may result in a level of regulation of the antibody response.

TSH has been shown to bind to B-lymphocytes, monocytes, and neutrophils presumably through TSH-like receptors since the receptors are coupled to cyclic AMP (cAMP; Chabaud and Lissiztsky 1977; Pekonen and Weintraub 1978; Harbour et al. 1990a, b). These receptors have binding characteristics which resemble one of the classical pituitary TSH receptors, but they are probably not classical TSH receptors (Coutelier et al. 1990). There is some evidence to suggest that TSH affects the cAMP levels, proliferation of and antibody release in human B-lymphocyte lines, and mitogen-stimulated B-lymphocyte populations from mouse spleens (Harbour et al. 1990a). These effects occur presumably through the TSH-type receptors which are present only on stimulated, but not resting, B-cells. This postulate is supported by the finding that normal resting human peripheral blood leukocytes do not bind TSH and have no TSH-induced increase in cAMP. Individuals with an active autoimmune response (Graves' disease or Hashimoto's disease, both forms of autoimmune thyroiditis) have elevated levels of TSH-type binding sites and show significant elevations in cAMP when stimulated with various concentrations of TSH (Harbour et al. 1990b, and unpublished observations by A. Minigutti, S. Leon, C. Keating, and D. Harbour, 1992). It can be postulated that levels of bioactive TSH-type binding sites on normal resting B-cells are not detectable, which prevents B-cells from responding to circulating levels of TSH (Harbour et al. 1990a). It is only when these levels are upregulated during activation that the B-cells are capable of a bioactive cAMP response to TSH (Harbour et al. 1990b).

Peripheral Sources of TRH

TRH has numerous extrahypothalamic sites of production and action. In mammals, TRH is found in many areas of the body. The extrahypothalamic localization includes numerous areas of the CNS (Spindel and Wurtman 1980). The forebrain, brain stem, posterior cortex, and cerebellum all contain detectable nanogram quantities of TRH. The pancreas of the neonatal rat contains very high TRH levels, localized to the islets of Langerhans (Moltz et al. 1977). These levels of TRH decline with age as the hypothalamic TRH increases. Removal of the pancreas in the 5-day-old rat results in a significant decline in plasma TRH by 3 h. In contrast, when the hypothalamus and extrahypothalamic forebrain are removed, plasma TRH levels are not changed after 3 h. Taken together, this evidence has led some researchers to speculate that the peripheral TRH does not come from the CNS but from the periphery itself and is probably synthesized within peripheral organs (Morley et al. 1977; Engler et al. 1981; Emerson 1986).

The neonate stomach and caecum also contain high levels, up to 3–4 ng, of irTRH (Engler et al. 1981). Normal circulating levels of TRH range from 6 to 16 pg/ml, but even these low levels are rapidly degraded by TRH-degrading enzymes in plasma. TRH is distributed in very high concentrations in the adult rat brain, 13.2 ng total, but it crosses the blood-brain barrier poorly and is rapidly degraded in plasma. Therefore, the presence of high, bioactive quantities in peripheral tissues provides important peripheral sources of TRH. There is evidence that the TRH precursor occurs in basal-granulated cell types of the GI tract (Fujita and Kobayashi 1981). Morley and coworkers (1977) have expressed the view that production of TRH by the GI tract and pancreas is not surprising since these sites are the major sources of circulating insulin, glucagon, somatostatin, vasoactive intestinal peptide (VIP), and bombesin peptides. The reproductive organs, the ovary, oviducts, uterus, prostate, testes, and seminal vesicles, contain large quantities of irTRH. In addition, the spleen contains measurable quantities of the TRH precursor, strongly suggesting that TRH may be produced in this tissue (Simard et al. 1989). There has been no thorough study of whether gut-associated lymphoid tissue produces the TRH or its precursor. The finding of the precursor in the spleen suggests the experiments to determine the cell source of synthesis in peripheral tissues.

Direct and Indirect Immunomodulatory Effects of Peripheral TRH

In addition to its indirect effect via the neuroendocrine pathway, peripheral TRH influences immune processes directly and indirectly. The aforementioned anatomical areas contain lymphoid tissue and other cells of the inflammatory response. TRH influences cells of the inflammatory response in a paracrine fashion, i.e., in a microenvironmental milieu. The result may be a significant localized immune response.

In mammals, several direct effects of TRH have been reported (Emerson 1986). It antagonizes sedatives, stimulates CNS and respiratory activities, elevates blood pressure, and regulates feeding behavior and body temperature. TRH also has potent behavioral effects.

Indirect peripheral effects include contraction and, in some cases, relaxation of smooth muscle cells. These effects occur either through TRH-stimulated release of histamine or acetylcholine. TRH has inhibitory effects on the secretion of gastric acid, pepsin and several pancreatic enzymes. Alteration of these physiologic processes may have potent effects on the overall immune response. Another example of an indirect effect of TRH not mediated via the neuroendocrine axis is its modulation of the various neurotransmitters, including serotonin, acetylcholine, and the catecholamines, dopamine, epinephrine, and norepinephrine, all of which have immunomodulatory activities (O'Dorosio and Panerai 1990). The plethora of activities of TRH both peripherally and centrally may explain its role in antagonizing endotoxin shock, a pathophysiologic response which is orchestrated by a cascade of mediators, many of which come from the immune system (for review see Harbour et al. 1991a, b). Therefore, TRH may have an indirect role in defense of the body from foreign invaders, such as infectious agents.

There is mounting evidence that TRH directly modulates the immune system. TRH has been reported to bind to membrane receptors, enhance inositol trisphosphate, and result in release of T-cell derived TSH (Harbour et al. 1988, 1989, 1990a). Kruger et al. (1989) reported that TRH enhances the in vitro plaque-forming cell (PFC) assay, which is reversed by antibody to TSH. However, it can be postulated that the mechanism of PFC enhancement is by inducing the production of the several lymphocyte-derived cytokines important in regulating B-cell response. In addition to the stimulation of the TSH intermediate, evidence shows that TRH stimulates the production and release of interleukin-2 (IL-2) at the protein and mRNA levels and of biologically active interferon-γ (IFN-γ) levels. TRH has no effect on IL-4 release. The enhanced antibody response can be abrogated by pretreatment of TSH with antibody to TSH and antibody to IFN-γ (Kruger et al. 1990; Harbour and Hughes 1991). The enhanced IFN-γ effect (as measured by antiviral activity) is abrogated by either antibody to IFN-γ or antibody to TRH (Harbour and Hughes 1991; Harbour et al. 1991b). Additionally, TRH has been reported to reconstitute an atrophied thymus and enhance in vivo antibody response, possibly by direct interaction with T-lymphocytes (Pierpaoli and Sorkin 1972; Pierpaoli and Xi 1990).

Summary of TRH Immunomodulatory Activity

The discussion above illustrates the pluripotential ability of TRH to alter the immune response. There are additional data from in vivo experiments which lend credence to the aforementioned studies. TRH has been reported to reconstitute an atrophied thymus and to enhance in vivo antibody response possibly by direct interaction with T-lymphocytes (Pierpaoli and Sorjin 1972; Pierpaoli and Xi 1990). One plausible mechanism for these results may be the in vitro and in vivo evidence showing TRH binding T-lymphocyte receptors, activating second messengers, and releasing growth-inducing cytokines (Harbour et al. 1988, 1990c).

The ability of TRH to stimulate in vitro production and release of IL-2 and IFN-γ can be reproduced in vivo. Support for this postulate is provided by TRH induction tests performed in vivo on normal and thymectomized BALB/c inbred mice (age and sex matched). Serum levels of TSH measured by radioimmunoassay at 0, 30, and 60 min confirmed that the TRH tests were working, i.e., normal mice showed a significant (greater than five fold) increase in serum TSH levels. Spleen cells from the mice at all three time points were analyzed for cytoplasmic presence of IL-2 and IFN-γ by immunofluorescence (IF) with monoclonal antibodies. The IF in normal spleen cells was significantly decreased at 30 and 60 min, strongly suggesting that TRH elicits release of IL-2 and IFN-γ from these cells in vivo (Fig. 1). Thymectomized mice had low levels of the cytokines and no change in IF after the TRH. Analysis of the spleen cells for RNA levels of IL-2 showed the presence of IL-2 messenger RNA at all three time points in normal mice, but in somewhat decreased amount by 60 min, as standardized with actin mRNA. The spleen cells of thymectomized mice contained no significant amount of IL-2 mRNA (Harbour et al. 1992).

Another study suggests that individuals with a blunted (reduced) pituitary TSH response to exogenous TRH also have blunted leukocyte-derived TSH response to exogenous TRH (Halbreich and Liu 1988; Harbour et al. 1988, 1990c). The suggested mechanism for the pituitary effect is that the TRH receptors are downregulated or desensitized either through excess TRH production or by catecholamine neurotransmitters (Loosen 1985). This hypothesis has not been directly tested with thyrotropin cells of the pituitary; however, studies of TRH receptors on leukocytes from individuals showing normal or blunted leukocyte-derived TSH response to TRH show a strong correlation between downregulation of the leukocyte TRH receptor and a blunted TSH response to TRH (Harbour et al. 1990c). Figure 2 shows several of the sources of TRH and illustrates some of the effects of TRH on the immune response.

Vasoactive Intestinal Peptide

VIP functions as a neurotransmitter in the central and peripheral nervous tissue (Hökfelt et al. 1982; O'Dorisio 1990; O'Dorisio and Panerai 1990). Autoradiographic mapping studies suggest that VIP binding sites appeared relatively early

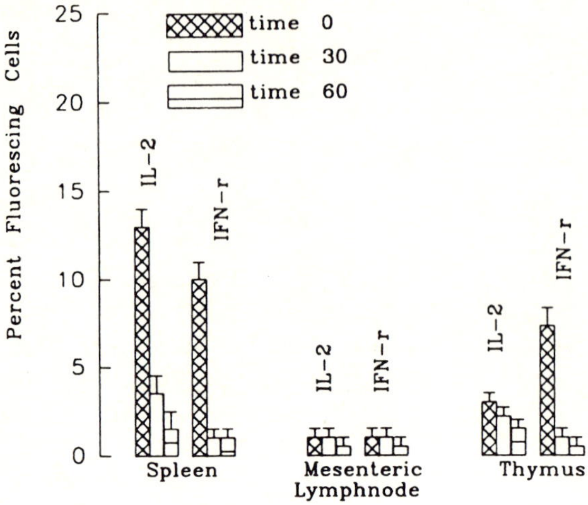

a

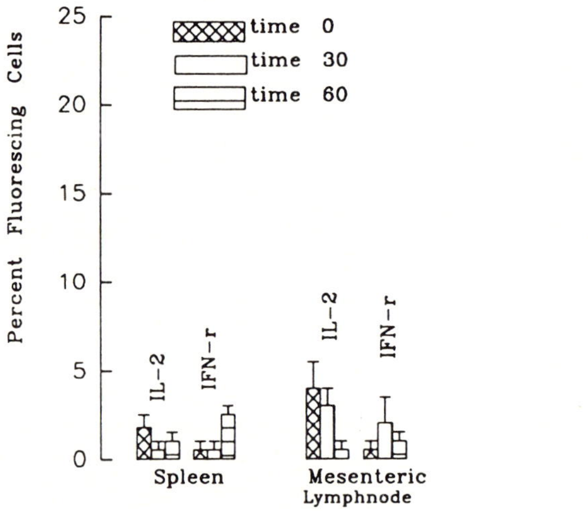

b

Fig. 1a, b. Effect of TRH on release of IL-2 and IFN-γ from lymphatic organs of normal (**a**) and thymectomized (**b**) mice in vivo. Note decrease in number of lymphoid cells showing immunofluorescence reaction to IL-2 and IFN-γ after exposure to TRH for 30 and 60 min

in the evolution of the vertebrate CNS (Dietl et al. 1990). VIP functions in a paracrine manner as a regulator of water and electrolyte secretion in the gut and of pancreatic secretion, as well as being a prolactin secretagogue (Schwartz et al. 1974; Yajima et al. 1986). VIP action on components of the immune system have been studied extensively. It has been shown to have broad activities over a wide range of immune effector cells (for review see O'Dorisio et al. 1981; Wenger et al. 1990). This is easily explained by the fact that many different subsets of immune effector cells express VIP receptors. VIP has been shown to indirectly

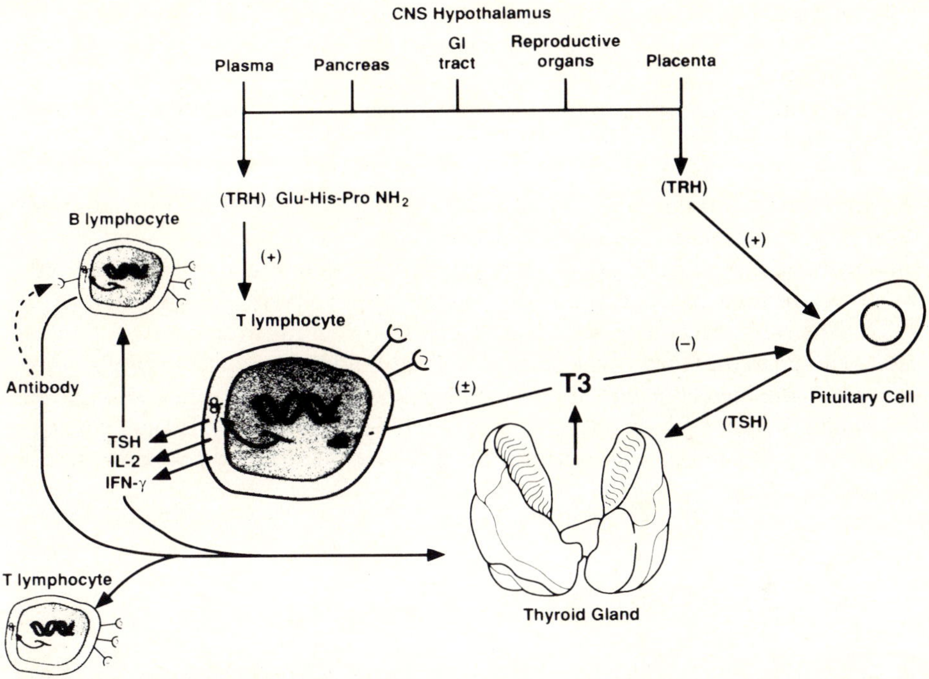

Fig. 2. Presumed interaction of TRH with the immune system. Direct effects of TRH from various cellular sources on the production and secretion of several cytokines by immune cells postulated to influence B-cell function (immunoglobulin), to enhance T-cell function, and to interact with the neuroendocrine system

suppress the proliferative response to mitogens by T-cells, presumably by inhibiting IL-2 production. VIP has been reported both to decrease and to enhance immunoglobulin synthesis (Krco et al. 1986). The peptide also inhibits NK cell activity, a process which can be reversed by preincubation of the cells with VIP. O'Dorisio (1986) postulated that the presence of VIP and VIP receptor positive cells in the gut-associated lymphoid tissue may be very important in regulating an immune response in the GI region.

Other investigators have postulated that VIP is produced by immunocytes, including reports of irVIP in mast cells, neutrophils, eosinophils, and leukemic basophils (Cutz et al. 1978; O'Dorisio et al. 1980). The immunoreactivity of VIP has been reported to be due to fragments of the intact molecule which bind to VIP receptors with agonist or antagonist activities depending on the piece of the fragment (Fournier et al. 1984; Goetzl et al. 1990). Another study reports VIP production in eosinophils found in granulomas formed around *Schistosoma mansoni* ova in liver and intestines. The importance of this VIP production is the modulation of the granuloma formation as a result of VIP inhibition of IL-2 synthesis and enhancement of IL-5 secretion (Blum et al. 1992). One of the more notable and significant actions of VIP appears to be its contributing to the homing of certain lymphocytes with high VIP receptor levels to the GI tract (Ottaway 1984).

The concept of hormonal milieu concentration is important since some neuropeptides and their receptors may play an active role in these processes and may be an important contributor to the homing mechanism of certain cells of the immune system (for review see O'Dorisio and Panerai 1990). For example, several investigators have shown that lymphocytes found in Peyer's patches of the gut have higher numbers of receptors for gut neuropeptides such as VIP, which are in high concentrations in these areas (for review see Ottaway 1984, 1987). The high levels may set up a concentration gradient allowing for these cells to home to that area of the peripheral lymphoid tissue. Another importance of hormonal milieu concentration is the response of the cell. It is not uncommon for bimodal responses to occur at pharmacologic versus physiologic concentrations (see also Janković and Marić, Stefano, and Scharrer and Stefano, in this volume).

Substance P and Other Tachykinins

These neuropeptides have been shown to be present in large amounts, not only within nervous tissue but also in immune organs such as the thymus, spleen, and those of the GI as well as in isolated immune cells (for review see McGillis et al. 1990). Some of these neuropeptides are released from nerve terminals which permeate lymphoid tissues throughout the mammalian body. Substance P (SP) is a member of a family of tachykinins which induce tachycardia and vasodilation most specifically by causing smooth muscle contraction and causing histamine release from mast cells. This type of activity makes SP an important mediator of hypersensitivity reactions. It is found in high concentrations in the intestinal tract and in mucosal and joint tissues. Other members of the family are substance K and neuromedin K. SP has the ability to enhance mitogenesis of human peripheral blood T-cells stimulated with the mitogens concanavalin A and phytohemagglutinin and mouse spleen cell responses to concanavalin A. SP also enhances T-cell dependent immunoglobulin (IgA and IgM) secretion in mesenteric lymph nodes and Peyer's patches (Payan and Goetzl 1983; Stanisz et al. 1986). In addition, SP has been reported to enhance cytotoxicity and lymphokine production in T-cells (McGillis et al. 1990). SP modulates several functions in macrophages in that tachykinins have been shown to stimulate IL-1, IL-6, and TNF-α in these cells (Lotz et al. 1988). It is chemotactic for human monocytes, and enhances numerous intracellular metabolites in these cells, such as arachadonic acid, leukotrienes and thromboxanes, mediators important for phagocytosis and peroxidase killing mechanisms (Ruff et al. 1985; Lotz et al. 1988). Additionally, presumably through these intracellular metabolites and also through the stimulation of phosphatidyl inositol metabolism, SP enhances the production of IL-1, IL-6, and tumor necrosis factor-α in macrophages (Hartung and Toyka 1983; Payan and Goetzl 1987).

Several investigators have evidence which strongly suggests that SP works in vivo by enhancing the inflammatory responses of rheumatoid arthritis in joint tissues (Lotz et al. 1987). One proposed mechanism whereby SP may mediate the increased inflammatory responses in arthritic joints is through an enhanced release of histamine by mast cells and via prostaglandin production. In fact, Bienenstock and coworkers (MacQueen et al. 1989) have shown that an enhanced mast cell response may be conditioned by use of classical conditioning techniques. These authors have proposed that the molecular mechanism whereby the enhanced mast cell activity occurs in arthritic joints is through the release of SP in the nerve terminals in the joint tissues. Elevated levels of SP have been detected in inflammatory exudates of arthritic joints in rats (Tissot et al. 1988). The resulting effect on the function of immunocytes migrating to an area of inflammation may be determined by the receptor expression and level of a particular neuropeptide released at the site of inflammation. Mast cells with SP receptors are attracted to areas of inflammatory joints with high concentrations of SP and cause damage to joint tissue by release of toxic metabolites.

This postulate becomes even more important when one considers that numerous cells of the immune system express high affinity (0.1–1 nM range) membrane receptors for SP (Hartung et al. 1986; Stanisz et al. 1987). These cells include mouse T- and B-cells of both spleen and Peyer's patch, macrophages, and possibly mast cells (MacQueen et al. 1989; McGillis et al. 1990). Another study showed that SP is produced by eosinophils within granulomas associated with *Schistosoma mansoni* in the murine model (Blum et al. 1992). The granulomatous response may be modulated by the finding that SP enhances IL-2 and IFN-γ secretion in this model. Although the majority of studies on the immunomodulatory activities of the tachykinins have been carried out with SP, the high degree of peptide homology between SP, substance K, and neuromedin K, and their cross-reactivity in receptor binding strongly suggest that all the tachykinins have diverse immunomodulatory activities most particularly in the peripheral immune response.

Bombesin, Neurotensin, and Neuropeptide Y

Neurotensin is a 13 amino acid peptide found in the CNS and in the gut. It is active in vitro at concentrations ranging from 10^{-14} to $10^{-9}\,M$ in enhancing phagocytosis, augmenting macrophage-mediated tumor cell killing, and enhancing lipopolysaccharide stimulated IL-1 production by macrophages (Bar-Shavit et al. 1982; Goldman et al. 1982; Bar-Shavit and Goldman 1990). There may be an interaction with and modulation of alveolar macrophage function in pulmonary disease since neurotensin nerve fibers are found in pulmonary tissues. Other investigators have reported enhanced phagocytosis of *Staphylococcus aureus* by neutrophils and increased Thy-1 antigen expression in adherant cells of the thymus (Molchanova et al. 1990). Neurotensin is another neuropeptide also found in invertebrates. Cells of the alimentary epithelium of *Branchiostoma* (amphioxi) react to antisera against mammalian neurotensin.

Bombesin is another neuropeptide widely distributed in the periphery but is present in very high concentrations in CNS tissue and gut tissues. The peptide has numerous regulatory functions, including thermoregulation, sensory transmission, gastric secretion, and food intake. Bombesin has been reported to have a role in cell proliferation and mitogenesis, particularly of lung epithelial cells, and it may be intricately involved in wound repair and healing (Wiedermann et al. 1988). It has also been reported to promote chemotaxis of human monocytes and activation of macrophages at very low concentrations (Hartung 1988). Another study reported that bombesin treatment significantly increases the phagocytic index in human monocytes and alveolar macrophages in normal subjects with an even higher index in individuals suffering from chronic bronchitis (Meloni et al. 1992). Certainly these cell types are very important in inflammatory responses and therefore would be pivotal characters in wound healing and repair.

Neuropeptide Y (NPY), a 36 amino acid peptide, is widely distributed in the CNS. It has been shown to be one of the peptides present in primary and secondary nerve fibers of the spleen (Fried et al. 1986). NPY is elevated after physical exercise and other forms of stress including heart failure and emotional stress (Lundberg et al. 1982, 1985; Pernow et al. 1986; Maisel et al. 1989; Castagne et al. 1987). Other investigators have demonstrated that NPY is elevated in lymphoid tissue, particularly spleen, after nerve stimulation (Lundberg et al. 1986, 1987). Except for its increase during times of stress, the influence of NPY on lymphoid tissues is unclear at this time. A recent paper by Irwin and coworkers (1991) has shown a close correlation between increased NPY, but not catecholamine levels, and significantly decreased NK cell activity in individuals suffering from clinical depression and those administering care to individuals with Alzheimer's disease.

Somatostatin

This neuropeptide is produced by both neuronal tissue and GI endocrine tissues in higher vertebrates and has been reported to occur in invertebrates (Barrington 1986) including the protozoan *Tetrahymena pyriformis* (Berelowitz et al. 1982). Several different somatostatin-related peptides, containing 14 and 28 amino acid residues, have been reported in animals from anglerfish to humans (McDonald et al. 1987). There have also been reports of somatostatin containing basophil cell lines (Goetzl et al. 1985), as well as its presence in the thymus (Lufgrens et al. 1984; Fuller and Verity 1989). Somatostatin appears to be inhibitory in nature. In the endocrine system it inhibits the release of insulin, growth hormone, thyroid hormones, and VIP (Reichlin 1986b). Somatostatin affects various immune functions, which include blocking of DNA and RNA synthesis in lymphoid and intestinal cells and inhibiting IgA in Peyer's patch lymphocytes (Payan et al. 1984; Stanisz et al. 1986; Newman et al. 1987). Blum et al. (1992) reported the presence of somatostatin 1–14 in murine granulomas formed around *S. mansoni* ova in liver and intestine. The somatostatin is produced by the granuloma macrophage. The report also shows somatostatin inhibition of IFN-γ production, therefore altering the course of the growth of the granuloma. As with other neuropeptides, the location of the somatostatin peptide and various receptor subtypes is fairly widespread throughout the brain, GI tissue, and lymphoid tissue, with different receptor subtypes expressed in various cell types, including the immune system (Bhathena and Recant 1980; Stead et al. 1987). In addition to the presence of various receptor subtypes, there is evidence that somatostatin may activate (or inhibit) multiple second messenger pathways (Jakobs et al. 1983; Martin et al. 1986; Aub et al. 1986). This may account for the differing effects of somatostatin on various cell types (for review see O'Dorisio 1990).

Vasopressin and Oxytocin

Oxytocin as well as vasopressin immunoreactivity in the thymus has been reported by several investigators (Geenen et al. 1986; Argiolas et al. 1990). At least one group has characterized the ir-oxytocin and found that its radioimmunoassay reactivity and HPLC retention time are almost identical with those of the synthetic oxytocin (Mellis et al. 1991). Additionally, the same group of investigators has found that immunosuppressant agents increase thymic ir-oxytocinlike activity. In particular, morphine tolerant/dependent rats were shown to have an increase in oxytocin immunoreactivity as a result of increased peptide production even though the thymus weight was decreased. These results are very intriguing in light of the early reports by Johnson and coworkers (1984) showing that vasopressin and oxytocin are able to replace the IL-2 requirement for antibody responses. In addition, vasopressin receptors have been found on human mononuclear cells (Elands et al. 1990). The presence of neuropeptides such as oxytocin and vasopressin in the thymus provides an alternative to the classical lymphokine requirement for initiation and perpetuation of an immune response (Geenan et al. 1988).

Luteinizing Hormone Releasing Hormone and Growth Hormone Releasing Hormone

Growth hormone releasing hormone (GHRH) protein and mRNA have been reported to be produced by rat spleen and thymus (Weigent and Blalock 1990a; Stephanou et al. 1991). One of the major proposed effects of GHRH on the immune system is actually indirect in that it induces the release of growth hormone (GH) by immunocytes with specific GHRH receptors (Weigant et al. 1990; Weigent and Blalock 1990b). GH has a general enhancing effect on the immune system much as does prolactin (for review see Kelley 1990; Weigent and Blalock 1990a). This activity includes increasing a proliferative response to mitogen, priming macrophages for superoxide production, and enhancing cytolytic and NK cell activity. Therefore, GHRH is certainly a potent immunomodulator, but through an indirect mechanism of regulating GH. As with GH, prolactin (stimulated by TRH) has a general enhancing effect on the majority of immune functions (for review see Roszman and Cross 1989; Bernton 1989). Prolactin has been shown to stimulate the expression of a network of growth related genes in T-cells, including c-*myc*, β-actin, ornithine decarboxylase, and an interferon regulatory factor-1 (Yu-Lee et al. 1990). Others have reported that prolactin must be internalized by the nucleus of the T-lymphocyte in order to enhance IL-2 stimulated proliferation (Clevenger et al. 1991). Finally, although GHRH and TRH have not yet been shown to induce lymphocyte-derived prolactin, the possibility, in light of its regulation of the pituitary prolactin gene, is intriguing. This is especially true in view of the data reported by investigators showing that concanavalin A stimulated murine spleen cells produce prolactinlike protein and mRNA (Kenner et al. 1988; for review see Bernton 1989).

Luteinizing hormone releasing hormone (LHRH) protein and an LHRH receptor produced by cells of the immune system have been isolated. Several groups have detected and characterized the LHRH protein in rat spleen and thymus by biochemical methods and have demonstrated bioactivity of the purified irLHRH (Emanuele et al. 1990; Marchetti et al. 1990; Azad et al. 1991a). Azad and coworkers showed an age-associated change in LHRH immunoreactivity. The level of irLHRH peaks during puberty, coinciding with gonadal maturation, and the irLHRH significantly declines in aged rats (Azad et al. 1991b). These data are consistent with previous findings of LHRH receptor sites in the rat thymus (Marchetti et al. 1989a). The latter result acquired in vivo significance when these investigators showed that LHRH agonists are able to increase reduced thymic weight, function, and LHRH binding sites in aged animals (Marchetti et al. 1989b).

This evidence shows that LHRH has direct immunomodulatory capacity, at least on the T-cell compartment, since LHRH agonists are able to enhance the proliferative capacity of thymocytes. This occurs presumably through LHRH receptors. In addition, LHRH acts indirectly; cells of the immune system produce ir-luteinizing hormone when stimulated in vitro with LHRH (Smith and Ebaugh 1990). Luteinizing hormone has immunomodulatory activity, as evidenced by its ability to enhance IL-1 and IL-2 release from thymocytes, to enhance the number of IgG and IgM PFCs and to increase the response to the mitogens concanavalin A and phytohemagglutinin in the presence of thymosin fraction 5 (Goldstein and Fritzler 1987; Rouabhia et al. 1987, 1991). In sum, LHRH and luteinizing hormone, regulated by LHRH, have a wide range of effects on the immune system.

Conclusions

This review provides evidence that the neuropeptides examined affect the immune system both in a direct and an indirect manner. These chemical messengers may act at close range, in which the concentration of the neuropeptide may be high, in paracrine and autocrine fashion, or in an endocrine manner, probably at lower concentrations, by interacting with their respective receptors. The response of the cell (or species) may take different forms depending on the message sent to direct the transcriptional and translational machinery involved in cellular growth regulators affecting proliferation and/or differentiation. These messages may be translated into other common mechanisms used by the immune system in inflammatory responses; chemoattraction, inhibition of migration, and activation or deactivation have all been described (for review see Roitt et al. 1989).

Since most of this chapter has focussed on TRH and its direct or indirect effects on immunomodulation both in vivo and in vitro, one final point needs to be emphasized. TRH is not restricted to vertebrates. TRH-like immunoreactivity has been demonstrated in an invertebrate, the snail *Lymnaea stagnalis*, and in a species of *amphioxi*, a prevertebrate (Jackson and Bolaffi 1983). In these species, TRH functions differently than in mammals in that there is no measurable release of neuroendocrine hormones after TRH administration (Grimm-Jørgensen and Voute 1979; Jackson 1981). One of the important roles of TRH in these species appears to be in regulating osmolarity. The finding of very high levels of TRH in amphibian skin is thought to play a physiologic role in the secretion of defensive substances or in the mechanisms of osmoregulation observed in these animals. Additionally, in amphibians, TRH appears to regulate prolactin secretion, indicating this function to be an early evolutionary event (Millar et al. 1983).

From an evolutionary standpoint the presence of TRH, along with many other chemical mediators, in the invertebrate system provides a rationale for postulating that this integrated system of a common language has been highly conserved (Martin 1990). Studying the invertebrate system allows us to observe, albeit somewhat reversed, how the primordial immune system has evolved from a simple system of mediators regulating behavior to one of a complex system with numerous functions, only one of which is specificity.

Finally, the finding of TRH throughout the body, its role in endotoxemia, respiratory tension, as well as its role in direct cellular communication with cells of the immune system argue that the more primitive functions of TRH have been retained. The TRH has expanded its primordial role only in the more complex vertebrate system.

Future study in this area may help to elucidate psychosomatic illness, the effects of stress and bereavement on predisposition to cancer, autoimmune disease, infectious disease, aging, and other body processes (Harbour and Blalock 1991). All of the neuropeptides mentioned in this chapter will be worth considering in these areas.

Acknowledgements. Some of the author's work reported in this chapter was supported by an NIH grant from the NINDS, NS 28069, and by the Department of Psychiatry and Behavioral Sciences, University of Texas Medical Branch, Galveston, Texas 77550, USA.

References

Argiolas A, Melis MR, Stancampiano R, Gessa GL (1990) Hypothalamic modulation of immunoreactive oxytocin in the rat thymus. Peptides 11:539–543

Aub DL, Frey EA, Sekura RD, Cate TE (1986) Coupling of the thyrotropin releasing hormone receptor to phospholipase C by a GTP binding protein distinct from the inhibitory or stimulatory GTP binding protein. J Biol Chem 261:933–941

Azad N, Emanuele NV, Halloran MM, Tentler J, Kelley MR (1991a) Presence of luteinizing hormone-releasing hormone (LHRH) mRNA in rat spleen lymphocytes. Endocrinology 128: 1679–1681

Azad N, Jurgens J, Young MR, Reda D, Duffner L, Kirsteins L, Emanuele NV, Lawrence AM (1991b) Presence of luteinizing hormone-releasing hormone in rat thymus. Prog Neuroendocrinology 4(2):113–120

Bar-Shavit Z, Goldman R (1990) Modulation of phagocyte activity by substance P and neurotensin. In: Freier S (ed) The neuroendocrine-immune Network. CRC Press, Boca Raton, pp 177–186

Bar-Schavit Z, Terry S, Blumberg S, Goldman R (1982) Neurotensin-macrophage interaction: specific binding and augmentation of phagocytosis. Neuropeptides 2:325–335

Barrington EJW (1986) The phylogeny of the endocrine system. Experentia 42:775–781

Berelowitz M, LeRoith D, VonSchenk H, Newgard C, Szabo M, Frohman LA, Shiloach J, Roth J (1982) Somatostatin-like immunoactivity and biological activity is present in T. pyriformis a ciliated protozoan. Endocrinology 110:1939–1944

Bernton EW (1989) Prolactin and immune host defense. Prog Neuroendocrinimmunol 2(1):21–29

Bhathena SJ, Recant L (1980) Somatostatin receptors on circulating human blood cells. Horm Metal Res 12:277–278

Blum AM, Metioali A, Mathew RC, Cook G, Elliott D, Weinstock JV (1992) Granuloma T lymphocytes in murine *Schistosoma mansoni* house somatostatin receptors and respond to somatostatin with decreased IGN-gamma secretion. J Immunology 149(11):3621–3626

Castagne V, Corder R, Gaillard R, Mormede P (1987) Stress-induced changes of circulating neuropeptide Y in the rat: comparison with catecholamines. Regul Pept 19:55–60

Chabaud O, Lissitzky S (1977) Thyrotropin specific binding to human peripheral blood monocytes and polymorphonuclear leukocytes. Mol Cell Endocrinol 7:79–86

Clevenger CV, Altman SW, Prystowsky MB (1991) Requirement for nuclear prolactin for interleukin-2-stimulated proliferation of T-lymphocytes. Science 253:77–79

Coutelier JP, Kehrl JH, Bellur SS, Kohn LD, Notkins AL, Prabhakar BS (1990) Binding and functional effects of thyroid stimulating hormone on human immune cells. J Clin Immunol 10(4):204–210

Cutz E, Chan W, Track NS, Goth A, Said S (1978) Release of vasoactive intestinal peptide in mast cells by histamine liberators. Nature 275:661–664

Dietl M, Hof P, Martin J, Magistretti P, Palacios J (1990) Autoradiographic analysis of the distribution of vasoactive intestinal peptide binding sites in the vertebrate nervous system: a phylogenetic study. J Endocrinol 502(1-2):14–26

Elands J, Van-Woudenberg A, Resink A, deKloet ER (1990) Vasopressin receptor capacity of human peripheral mononuclear cells is sex dependent. Brain behav Immun 4(1):30–38

Emanuele NV, Emanuele MA, Tentler J, Kirsteins L, Azad N, Lawrence AM (1990) Rat spleen lymphocytes contain an immunoactive and bioactive luteinizing hormone-releasing hormone. Endocrinology 126:2482–2486

Emerson CH (1986) Extrapituitary effect of thyrotropin releasing hormone. In: Ingbar SH, Braverman LE (eds) The thyroid: a fundamental and clinical text. Lippincott, Philadelphia, pp 1472–1489

Engler D, Scanlon MF, Jackson IMD (1981) Thyrotropin releasing hormone in the systemic circulation is derived from the pancreas and other extraneural tissues. J Clin Invest 67:800–808

Fournier A, Saunders JK, St Pierre S (1984) Synthesis, conformational studies and biological activities of VIP and related fragments. Peptides 5:169–177

Fried G, Terenius L, Brodin E, Efendic S, Dockray G, Fahrenkrug J, Goldstein M, Hökfelt T (1986) Neuropeptide Y, enkephalin and noradrenaline coexist in sympathetic neurons innervating the bovine spleen. Biochemical and immunohistochemical evidence. Cell Tissue Res 243:495–508

Fujita T, Kobayashi S (1981) The endocrine cell. In: Bloom SR, Polak JM (eds) Gut hormones. Churchill Livingston, Edinburgh, pp 90–95

Fuller PJ, Verity K (1989) Somatostatin gene expression in the thymus gland. J Immunol 143:1015–1017

Geenan V, Legros JJ, Franchimont P, Baudrihaye M, Defresne MP, Boniver J (1986) The neuroendocrine thymus: coexistence of oxytocin and neurophysin in the human thymus. Science 232:208–210

Geenan V, Defresne MP, Robert F, Legros JJ, Franchimont P, Boniver J (1988) The neurohormonal thymic microenvironment: immunocytochemical evidence that thymic nurse cells are neuroendocrine cells. Neuroendocrinology 47:365–368

Goetzl EJ, Chernov-Rogan T, Cookee MP, Renold F, Payan DG (1985) Endogenous somatostatin-like peptides of rat basophilic leukemia cells. J Immunol 135:2707–2712

Goetzl EJ, Grotmol T, Van Dyke RW, Turck CW, Wershil B, Galli SJ, Sreedharan SP (1990) Generation and recognition of vasoactive intestinal peptide by cells of the immune system. In: O'Dorisio MS, Panerai A (eds) Neuropeptides and immunopeptides: messengers in a neuro-immune axis. Ann NY Acad Sci 594: 34–44

Goldman R, Bar-Shavit Z, Shazen E, Terry S, Blumberg S (1982) Enhancement of phagocytosis by neurotensin, a newly found biological activity of the neuropeptide. In: Normann SJ, Sorkin E (eds) Macrophages and natural killer cells: regulation and function. Plenum, New York, pp 133–141

Goldstein EJ, Fritzer MJ (1987) The role of the thymus-hypothalamic-pituitary-gonadal axis in normal immune processes and autoimmunity. J Rheumatol 14:982–990

Grimm-Jørgensen Y, Voute CL (1979) A possible role of thyrotropin releasing hormone in the seasonal adaptation of salt transport in the frog. Gen Comp Endocrinol 37:482–486

Halbreich U, Liu X (1989) In vitro ir-TSH response of mononuclear leukocytes to TRH in normal women and depressed patients – relationship to in vivo TRH tests. Am College Neurophychopharmacology Meeting Abstracts p 183

Harbour DV, Blalock JE (1991) Interactions of other systems with the immune system. In: Coulam CB, Faulk WP, McIntyre J (eds) Immunological obstetrics. Norton, New York (in press)

Harbour DV, Hughes TK (1991) Thyrotropin releasing hormone (TRH) induces gamma interferon release. FASEB J Abstracts 75th annual meeting. Abstract no 5884, pA1385

Harbour DV, Anderson A, Farrington J, Wassef A, Smith EM, Meyer WJ (1988) Decreased mononuclear leukocyte TSH responsiveness in patients with major depression. Biol Psychiatry 23:797–806

Harbour DV, Kruger T, Coppenhaver D, Smith EM, Meyer WJ (1989) Differential expression and regulation of thyrotropin (TSH) in T-cell lines. Mol Cell Endocrinol 64:229–241

Harbour DV, Leon S, Keating C, Hughes TK (1990a) Thyrotropin (TSH) modulates B-cell function through specific bioactive receptors. Prog NeuroEndocrinImmunol 3(4):266–276

Harbour DV, Leon S, Keating C, Dallas J (1990b) Role of B-cell thyrotropin receptors in autoimmune disease. 5th annual conference on clinical immunology. Chicago, abstract no 74

Harbour DV, Smith EM, Meyer WJ (1990c) The thyrotropin releasing hormone induced pituitary thyroid stimulating hormone response correlates with the TRH induced leukocyte TSH response. Ann NY Acad Sci 594:385–387

Harbour DV, Galin FS, Hughes TK, Smith EM, Blalock JE (1991a) Role of leukocyte-derived pro-opiomelanocortin peptides in endotoxic shock. Circ Shock 35(3):181–191

Harbour DV, Van Cleave CL, Kulvecki AD (1991b) Thyrotropin releasing hormone receptors (TRH) elicit the release of multiple cytokines from lymphoid cells. Clin Immunol Soc Atlanta, abstract no 12

Harbour DV, Jyoti M, Kang WL, Kulvecki A (1992) Evidence for an in vivo hypothalamic-lymphoid-thyroid axis. Endocrine Society 74th annual meeting, San Antonio. Abstract no 442, 162

Hartung HP (1988) Activation of macrophages by neuropeptides. Brain Behav Immun 2:275–281

Hartung HP, Toyka KV (1983) Activation of macrophages by substance P: induction of oxidative burst and thromboxane release. Eur J Pharmacol 89:301–305

Hartung HP, Wolters K, Toyka K (1986) Substance P: binding properties and studies on cellular responses in guinea pig macrophages. J Immunol 136:3856–3863

Hökfelt T, Schultzbert M, Lundberg JM, Fuxe K, Mutt V, Fahrenkrug J, Said SI (1982) Distribution of vasoactive intestinal polypeptide in the central and peripheral nervous systems as revealed by immunochemistry. In: Said SI (ed) Vasoactive intestinal peptide advances in peptide hormone research series. Raven, New York, pp 65–79

Ingbar SH, Braverman LE (eds) (1986) The thyroid: a fundamental and clinical text. Lippincott, Philadelphia

Irwin M, Brown M, Patterson T, Hauger R, Mascovich A, Grant I (1991) Neuropeptide Y and natural killer cell activity: findings in depression and Alzheimer caretaker stress. FASEB J 5(15):3100

Jackson IMD (1981) Evolutionary significance of the phylogenetic distribution of the mammalian hypothalamic releasing hormones. Fed Proc 40:2545–2552

Jackson IMD, Bolaffi J (1983) Phylogenetic distribution of TRH: significance and function. In: Griffiths EL, Bennett GW (eds) Thyrotropin releasing hormones. Raven, New York, pp 191–202

Jackson IMD, Reichlin S (1974) Thyrotropin-releasing hormone (TRH): distribution in hypothalamic and extrahypothalamic brain tissues of mammalian and submammalian chordates. Endocrinology 95:854–862

Jakobs KH, Aktories K, Schultz G (1983) A nucleotide regulatory site for somatostatin inhibition by adrenylate cyclase in S49 lymphoma cells. Nature 303:177–178

Johnson HM, Farrar WL, Torren BA (1984) Vasopressin replacement of interleukin-2 requirement in gamma interferon production: lymphokine activity of a neuroendocrine hormone. J Immunol 129:(3)983–986

Kelley KW (1990) The role of growth hormone in modulation of the immune response. Ann NY Acad Sci 594:95–103

Kenner J, Smith P, Bernton E, Hartmann D, Holaday J (1988) Murine splenic lymphocytes demonstrate con. A inducible PRL-like immunoreactivity as determined by immunocytochemistry. 18th annual metting, Soc Neurosci Abstr 756

Krco CJ, Gores A, Go VL (1986) Gastrointestinal regulatory peptides modulate in vitro immune reactions of mouse lymphoid cells. Clin Immunol Immunopathol 39(2):308–318

Kruger TE, Blalock JE (1986) Cellular requirements for thyrotropin enhancement of in vitro antibody production. J Immunol 137:197–201

Kruger T, Smith LR, Harbour DV, Blalock JE (1990) Thyrotropin: an endogenous regulator of the in vitro immune response. J Immunol 142:744–750

Loosen PT (1985) The TRH-induced TSH response in psychiatric patients: a possible neuroendocrine marker. Psychiatric Review 10(3):237–260

Lotz M, Carson DA, Vaughn JH (1987) Substance P activation of rheumatoid synoviocytes: neural pathway in pathogenesis of arthritis. Science 235:893–895

Lotz M, Vaughn JH, Carson DA (1988) Effects of neuropeptides on production of inflammatory cytokines by human monocytes. Science 241:1218–1221

Lufgrens I, Revhaug A, Burhol PG, Giercksky KE, Jenssen TG (1984) Vasoactive intestinal polypeptide and somatostatin in leukocytes. Scand J Clin Lab Invest 44:347–351

Lundberg JM, Terenius L, Hökfelt T, Martinsson CR, Tatemoto K, Mutt V, Polak J, Bloom S, Goldstein M (1982) Neuropeptide Y (NPY)-like immunoreactivity in peripheral noradrenergic neurons and effects of NPY on sympathetic function. Acta Physiol Scand 116:477–480

Lundberg JM, Martinsson A, Hemsen A, Theodorsson-Norheim E, Svendenhag J, Ekblom B, Hjemdahl P (1985) Co-release of neuropeptide Y and catecholamines during physical exercise in man. Biochem Biophys Res Commun 133:30–36

Lundberg JM, Rudehill A, Sollevi A, Theodorsson-Norheim E, Hamberger B (1986) Frequency- and reserpine-dependent chemical coding of sympathetic transmission: differential release of noradrenaline and neuropeptide Y from pig spleen. Neurosci Lett 63:96–100

Lundberg JM, Pernow J, Fried G, Anggard A (1987) Neuropeptide Y and noradrenaline mechanisms in relation to reserpine induced impairment of sympathetic neurotransmission in the cat spleen. Acta Physiol Scand 131:1–10

MacQueen G, Marshall J, Perdue M, Siegel S, Bienenstock J (1989) Pavlovian conditioning of rat mucosal mast cells to secrete rat mast cell protease II. Science 243:83–85

Maisel AS, Scott NA, Motulsky HJ, Michel MC, Boublik JH, Rivier JE, Ziegler M, Allen RK, Brown MR (1989) Elevation of plasma neuropeptide Y levels in congestive heart failure. Am J Med 86:43–48

Marchetti B, Guarcello V, Morale MC, Bartoloni G, Farinella Z, Cordaro S, Scapagnini U (1989a) Luteinizing hormone-releasing hormone-binding sites in the rat thymus: characteristics and biological function. Endocrinology 125:1025–1036

Marchetti B, Guarcello V, Morale MC, Bartoloni G, Raiti F, Palumbo G Jr, Farinella Z, Cordaro S, Scapagnini U (1989b) Luteinizing hormore-releasing hormone (LHRH) agonist restoration of age-associated decline of thymus weight, thymic LHRH receptors, and thymocyte proliferative capacity. Endocrinology 125:1037–1045

Marchetti B, Maier CC, LeBoeuf RD, Blalock JE (1990) Luteinizing hormone-releasing hormone gene expression in the thymus. Society for Neuroscience. 20th annual meeting, St Louis. Abstract p 1206

Martin JB (1990) On the economy of the biological systems. Prog NeuroEndocrinImmunol 3:ii

Martin TF, Lucas DO, Bajjalich SM, Kowalchyk JA (1986) Thyrotropin-releasing hormone activates a Ca^{2+} dependent polyphosphoinositide phosphodiesterase in permeable GH_3 cells. J Biol Chem 261:2981–2992

McDonald JK, Greimer F, Bauer GE, Elde RP, Noe BD (1987) Separate cell types that express two different forms of somatostatin in anglerfish islets can be immunohistochemically differentiated. J Histochem Cytochem 35(2):155–162

McGillis JP, Mitsuhashi M, Payan DG (1990) Immunomodulation by tachykinin neuropeptides. Ann NY Acad Sci 594:85–94

Mellis MR, Stancampiano R, Devoto P, Gessa GL, Argiolas A (1991) Thymic oxytocin-like immunoreactivity is increased in morphine tolerrant rats. Prog NeuroEndocrinImmunol 4:106–112

Meloni F, Bertoletti R, Corsico A, Di Frazio P, Cecchettin M, Gialdroni-Grassi G (1992) Bombesin-gastrin releasing peptide levels of peripheral mononuclear cells, monocytes and alveolar macrophages in chronic bronchitis. Int J Tissue Reaction 14(4): 195–201

Millar RP, Nicholson S, King JA, Louw GN (1983) Functional significance of TRH in metamorphing and adult anurans. In: Griffiths EC, Bennett GW (eds) Thyrotropin releasing hormones. Raven, New York, pp 127–227

Molchanova IV, Belokrylov GA, Popova O (1990) Neurotensin, cholecystokinin octapeptide and pentagastrin as immunogenesis regulators. 1st international congress ISNIM. Workship on neuroimmunomodulation. Abstract 130, p 192

Moltz JH, Dobbs BE, McCann SM, Gawcett CP (1977) Hypothalamic substances effect release of glucagon from islets of Langerhans. Endocrinology 101:196–202

Morley JE, Garven TJ, Pekary AE, Hershman JM (1977) Thyrotropin-releasing hormone in the gastrointestinal tract. Biochem Biophys Res Commun 79:314–318

Newman JB, Luis F, Townsend CM (1987) Somatostatin. In: Thompson C, Greeley GH, Rayford PL, Townsend CM (eds) Gastrointestinal Endocrinology. McGraw-Hill, New York, Chap 21

O'Dorisio MS (1986) Neuropeptides and gastrointestinal immunity. Am J Med 81:74–84

O'Dorisio MS (1990) The role of substance P, somatostatin and vasoactive intestinal peptide in modulation of mucosal immunity. In: Freier S (ed) The neuroendocrine immune network. CRC Press, Boca Raton, pp 187–198

O'Dorisio MS, Panerai A (eds) (1990) Neuropeptides and immunopeptides: messengers in a neuroimmune axis. Ann NY Acad Sci 594

O'Dorisio MS, O'Dorisio TM, Cataland S, Balcerazak SP (1980) Vasoactive intestinal peptide as a biochemical marker for polymorphonuclear leukocytes. J Lab Clin Med 96:666–672

O'Dorisio MS, Hermina N, Balcerzak SP, O' Dorisio TM (1981) Vasoactive intestinal peptide stimulation of adenylate cyclase in purified human leukocytes. J Immunol 127:2551–2554

Ottaway CA (1984) In vitro alteration of receptors for vasoactive intestinal peptide changes in the in vivo localization of mouse T cells. J Exp Med 160:1054–1069

Ottaway CA (1987) Selective effects of VIP on the mitogenic response of murine T cells. Immunology 62:291–297

Payan DG, Goetzl EJ (1983) Specific stimulation of human T-lymphocytes in pulmonary inflammation. J Immunol 131:1613–1615

Payan DG, Goetzl EJ (1987) Substance P receptor-dependent responses of leukocytes in pulmonary inflammation. Annu Rev Respir Dis 136:539–543

Payan DG, Hess CA, Goetzl EJ (1984) Inhibition by somatostatin of the proliferation of T-lymphocytes and Molt 4B lymphoblasts. Cell Immunol 84:433–438

Pernow J, Lundberg JM, Kaijser L, Hjemdahl P, Theodorsson-Norheim E, Martinsson A, Pernow B (1986) Plasma neuropeptide Y-like immunoreactivity and catecholamines during various degrees of symphathetic activation in man. Clin Physiol 6:561–578

Pierpaoli W, Sorkin E (1972) Role of the thymus in programming in mice with congenital absence of thymus. Nature 238:282–284

Pierpaoli W, Xi C (1990) The involvement of pineal gland and melatonin in immunity and aging. I Thymus mediated, immuno-reconstituting and antiviral activity of thyrotropin releasing hormone. J Neuroimmunol 27:99–109

Pekonen F, Weintraub BD (1979) Thyrotropin receptors on bovine thyroid membranes: two types with different affinities and specificities. Endocrinology 105(2):352–359

Provinciali M, Fabris N (1990) Modulation of lymphoid cell sensitivity to interferon by thyroid hormones. J Endocrinol Invest 13:107–112

Reichlin S (1986a) Neuroendocrine control of thyrotropin secretion. In: Ingbar SH, Braverman LE (eds) The thyroid: a fundamental and clinical text. Lippincott, Philadelphia, pp 241– 266

Reichlin S (1986b) Somatostatin: historical aspects. Scand J Gastroenterol Suppl 199: 1–10

Roitt IM, Brostoff J, Male Dk (1989) Immunology. Harper and Row, New York

Roszman TL, Cross RJ (1989) Neuroendocrine modulation of immune function. The role of prolactin. Prog NeuroEndocrinImmunol 2(1):17–20

Rouabhia M, Ghanmi Z, Deschaux P (1987) Luteotrophic hormone: receptor and inhibition of T-cytotoxicity in vitro. Perspect Biol 89:119–126

Rouabhia M, Chakir J, Deschaux P (1991) Interaction between the immune and endocrine systems: immune modulatory effects of luteinizing hormone. Prog NeuroEndocrinImmunol 4(2):86–91

Ruff MR, Wahl SM, Pert CB (1985) Substance P receptor mediated chemotaxis of human monocytes. Peptides 2 [Suppl 6] 107–111

Schwartz CJ, Kimberg DV, Sheerin HE, Field M, Said SI (1974) Vasoactive intestinal peptide stimulation of adenylate cyclase and active electrolyte secretion in intestinal mucosa. J Clin Invest 51:536–543

Simard M, Pekary AE, Smith VP, Hershman JM (1989) Thyroid hormones modulate thyrotropin releasing hormone biosynthesis in tissues outside the hypothalamic pituitary axis of male rats. Endocrinology 125:524–531

Smith EM, Ebaugh MJ (1990) Luteogenic activity from human leukocytes. Ann NY Acad Sci 594:492–493

Spindel ER, Wurtman RJ (1980) TRH immunoreactivity in rat brain regions, spinal cord and pancreas: validation by high pressure liquid chromatography. Brain Res 201:279–288

Stanisz AM, Befus D, Bienenstock J (1986) Differential effects of vasoactive intestinal peptide, substance P and somatostatin on immunoglobulin synthesis and proliferation by lymphocytes from Peyer's patches, mesenteric lympth nodes and spleen. J Immunol 136:152–156

Stanisz AM, Scicchitano R, Dazin P, Bienenstock J, Payan DG (1987) Distribution of substance P receptors on murine spleen and Peyer's patch T- and B-cells. J Immunol 139:1613–1615

Stead RH, Bienenstock J, Stanisy AM (1987) Neuropeptide regulation of mucosal immunity. Immunol Rev 100:333–359

Stephanou A, Knight RA, Lightman SL (1991) Production of a growth hormone releasing hormone-like peptide and its mRNA by human lymphocytes. Neuroendocrinology 53:628–633

Stolc V (1972a) Inhibitory effect of pituitary factor on phagocytosis and iodine metabolism in human leukocytes. Endocrinology 91:835–842

Stolc V (1972b) Regulation of iodine metabolism in human leukocytes by adenine 3′5′-monophosphate. Biochem Biophys Res Commun 264:285–288

Tissot M, Pradelles P, Giroud JP (1988) Substance P-like levels in inflammatory exudates. Inflammation 12:25–30

Weigent DA, Blalock JE (1990a) Growth hormone releasing hormone production by rat leukocytes. Int Rev Immunol 4:193–204

Weigent DA, Blalock JE (1990b) Growth hormone and the immune system. Prog NeuroEndocrin-Immunol 3(4):231–241

Weigent DA, Baxter JB, Guarcello V, Blalock JE (1990) Growth hormone releasing hormone receptors in the rat immune system. Ann NY Acad Sci 594:432–434

Wenger GD, O'Dorisio MS, Goetzl EJ (1990) Vasoactive intestinal peptide messenger in a neuroimmune axis. In: O'Dorisio MS, Panerai A (eds) Neuropeptides and immunopeptides: messengers in a neuroimmune axis. Ann NY Acad Sci 594:104-119

Wiederman CJ, Ruff MR, Pert CB (1988) Bombesin peptides: neuropeptides with mitogenic activity. Brain Behav Immunol 2(4):301–310

Yajima Y, Akita Y, Saito T (1986) Pertussis toxin blocks the inhibitory effects of somatostatin on cAMP-dependent vasoactive intestine peptide and cAMP-independent thyrotropin releasing hormone-stimulated prolactin of GH_3 cells. J Biol Chem 261:2684–2689

Yu-Lee LY, Stevens AM, Hrachovy JA, Schwarz LA (1990) Prolactin- mediated gene regulation of gene transcription in lymphocytes. Ann NY Acad Sci 594: 146–155

Enkephalins as Regulators of Inflammatory Immune Reactions

B. D. Janković[1] and D. Marić[1]

Introduction

Inflammation is a complex reaction of living tissue which tends to eliminate injurious agents and to repair damaged tissue. Early observations of inflammation showed (a) vascular changes (Virchow 1858), (b) local circulatory disturbances including margination and stacking of leukocytes and their migration through the vascular wall (Cohnheim 1867), and (c) phagocytic elimination of inflammatory agents (Metchnikoff 1893). In 1923 Rossle advanced the concept of "allergic inflammation" as the inflammatory reaction that follows interaction between foreign protein or antigen and antibody in an animal which had previously been in contact with that particular antigen. Studies of inflammation revealed an initial local alteration of cells and tissues (Schade 1923). Lewis (1927) presented evidence that vascular phenomena of the inflammatory reaction are initiated by histamine or other mediators. Menkin (1940) isolated thermolabile and thermostable substances from inflammatory exudates which caused an increase in vascular permeability and emigration of leukocytes. The important observation of Enrich (1956) that inflammatory vascular changes may be induced by certain neurogenic factors stimulated the search for other mediators, regulators, and modulators involved in mechanisms underlying the inflammatory reaction.

The old "humoral" concept of inflammation is now being reexamined by cooperative efforts of biochemists, cell biologists, pharmacologists, pathophysiologists, and immunologists, aided by superior modern technology. A wide range of methodologies and in vivo and in vitro models have been employed to elucidate the body's most important adaptive/defensive responses to a variety of intrinsic and extrinsic insults. This chapter deals with the effects of intraperitoneally administered opioid pentapeptides, the enkephalins, on immunologically induced inflammatory reactions.

Inflammatory Reactions: Mechanisms

The three principal components of inflammation are increases in (a) blood flow to the affected area, (b) capillary permeability in the local vasculature, caused by retraction of the endothelial cells which allows passage of larger serum molecules

[1] Immunology Research Center, Vojvode Stepe 458, 11221 Belgrade, Yugoslavia

Scharrer et al. (Eds.)
Neuropeptides and Immunoregulation

and various biologically active mediators into the interstitial space, and (c) migration of cells guided to the inflammatory area by chemotactic stimuli. The cell types seen in different inflammatory foci vary widely depending on the nature of the stimulus, its persistence, and the reacton that it elicits. They may include polymorphonuclear neutrophils (PMN; Spisani and Traniello 1979), eosinophils (Goetzl 1977), basophils (Conroy et al. 1977), mast cells (Sullivan and Parker 1976), platelets (Nachman and Polley 1979), macrophages (Spector 1979), and in the case of antigenic stimuli mononuclear cells (Dvorak et al. 1974). Furthermore, various types of inflammatory reactions are complicated by the involvement of several other factors collectively termed "amplification systems" (Wells 1982). The pathophysiology of these mediators in inflammatory reactions is the subject of several comprehensive reviews (Movat 1971; Macfarlane 1973; Wilhelm 1973; Willoughby 1973; Weissman et al. 1979; Henson and Murphy 1989).

Various neuropeptides are involved in inflammatory processes: vasoactive intestinal peptide (Morice et al. 1983), neurotensin (Foreman et al. 1982), somatostatin (Theoharides and Douglas 1981; Goetzl and Payan 1984), substance P (Hagermark et al. 1978; Payan et al. 1984; Pernow 1985), gastrin (Tharp et al. 1984), and the opioid peptides (Carr et al. 1982; Yamasaki et al. 1983; Casale et al. 1984). Here, we consider mainly the interrelationship between the opioid system and immunoinflammatory reactions.

Opioid Peptides as Immunomodulatory Agents

By definition, opioid peptides are substances that simulate pharmacological, effects of morphine and similar opiates. The family of opioid peptides contains about 40 members, including enkephalins (Hughes et al. 1975), endorphins (Goldstein 1976), dynorphins (Goldstein et al. 1979), and other opioid peptide chains of different lengths and amino acid sequences (Hedner and Cassuto 1987). Opioid peptides are derived from at least three polypeptide precursors, pro-opiomelanocortin, proenkephalin, and prodynorphin, which originate mainly in the adenohypophysis, adrenal medulla, and hypothalamic-neurohypopysial system, respectively (Numa 1984). A characteristic feature of opioid peptides is that they all contain one or more copies of the two simplest opioid pentapeptides: methionine-enkephalin (tyrosine-glycine-glycine-phenylalanine-methionine) and leucine-enkephalin (tyrosine-glycine-glycine-phenylalanine-leucine). The opioid peptides may specifically bind to at least four types of opioid receptors: μ, δ, κ, and ε, which are unevenly distributed in cells and tissues (Pert and Snyder 1973; Terenius 1973; Pearson et al. 1980; Valette et al. 1980; Kamikawa and Shima 1983). By interaction with one or more of these receptors, and depending on microenvironmental conditions, different opioid peptides exert a whole array of biological effects: analgesia (Cox et al. 1975; Loh et al. 1976), regulation of neurosecretion in the hypothalamus (Meites 1980), modulation of affective behavior (Atweh and Kuhar 1983), stimulation of sexual (Meyerson and Terenius

1977) and feeding behavior (Grandison and Guidotti 1977), and regulation of hypotension and hypothermia (Bloom et al. 1976). They play a role as neurotransmitters in the central and peripheral nervous systems (Beaumont and Hughes 1979), as modulators in mechanisms of stress (Guillemin et al. 1977; Madden et al. 1977; Rossier et al. 1977) in peristalsis (Kromer et al. 1981), intestinal function (Hedner and Cassuto 1987), and electrolyte transport (Dobbins et al. 1981).

Modulatory effects of Met-enkephalin and morphine have been shown on normal lymphocytes (Wybran et al. 1979) and lymphocytes of opiate addicts (McDonough et al. 1980). Opioid peptides modulate natural killer (NK) activity in the peripheral blood (Mathews et al. 1983; Faith et al. 1984; Kay et al. 1984) and spleen (Carr and Klimpel 1986). They induce alterations in leukocyte morphology (Falke and Fischer 1985; Scharrer and Stefano, this volume) suppress antibody production (Johnson et al. 1982; Heijnen et al. 1986) and stimulate proliferation of mononuclear cells (Gilman et al. 1982; Puppo et al. 1985) and the activity of suppressor lymphocytes (McCain et al. 1986). They elicit production of γ-interferon by mononuclear cells (Brown and Van Epps 1985; Mandler et al. 1986) and large granular lymphocytes of the peripheral blood (Mandler et al. 1986). They increase the activity of cytotoxic lymphocytes in mixed lymphocyte reaction (Carr and Klimpel 1986), IgG-dependent, antibody-dependent cellular cytotoxicity of macrophages (Foris et al. 1984), and the ability of neutrophils to adhere to various structures (Fischer and Falke 1984). Opioid peptides also modulate the respiration of mononuclear cells (Sharp et al. 1985).

Most of these immunomodulatory activities of opioid peptides can be blocked by opioid peptide antagonists, for example naloxone, indicating that they act through interaction with specific opioid receptors (Carr 1988; Stefano, this volume).

Immunocytes contain opioid receptors: μ and δ receptors are present on T- and B-lymphocytes (Mehrishi and Mills 1983; Smith et al. 1984) κ receptors on thymoma cell lines (Fiorica and Spector 1988) and ε receptors on the cell membranes of lymphocytes and thymoma cells after cultivation (Hazum et al. 1979; Schweigerer et al. 1985). Furthermore, cells of the immune system express genes encoding for opioid peptide precursors, namely proenkephalin (Zurawski et al. 1986; Monstein et al. 1986) and pro-opiomelanocortin (Lolait et al. 1986). Most probably immunocytes synthesize and secrete enkephalin (Felten et al. 1985) and β-endorphin (Lolait et al. 1984; Smith et al. 1986).

As to the role of opioids in inflammation, various types of allergic inflammatory reactions have been shown to be exacerbated or suppressed by different opioid peptides (Carr et al. 1982; Oyama et al. 1983; Amir and Ree 1985). In vitro, β-endorphin and Met-enkephalin were found to modulate the production of T-lymphocyte chemotactic factor (Brown and Van Epps 1985), which is known to attract these cells to inflammatory foci. These peptides themselves are potent chemotactic agents for different inflammatory cells such as peripheral blood lymphocytes (Van Epps and Saland 1984), monocytes (Ruff et al. 1985), and PMN (Simkins et al. 1984; Horvath et al. 1985; Scharrer and Stefano, this volume). Certain types of inflammatory cells, for example, mast cells, express on their plasma membrane at least one type of opioid receptor, and β-endorphin, dynorphin, and other opioids can specifically stimulate these cells to release different inflammatory mediators (Yamasaki et al. 1983; Casale et al. 1984). Opioid peptide receptors have also been found on monocytes (Lopker et al. 1980), PMN (Falke and Fischer 1985; Stefano, this volume), T-lymphocytes (Farrar et al. 1987), platelets (Mehrishi and Mills 1983), and endothelial cells of the vascular system (Feuerstein and Faden 1982; Boogaerts et al. 1983). Some of these inflammatory cells have also been shown to synthesize and secrete their own opioid peptide products. Met-enkephalin is present in platelets (Mosnaim et al. 1985) and T-cells (Zurawski et al. 1986), and β-endorphin in lymphocytes (Smith and Blalock 1981) and macrophages (Lolait et al. 1986).

The great majority of these studies deal with the role of opioid peptides by employing in vitro methods. By contrast, the authors' studies reported here refer exclusively to the in vivo effects of opioids on well-defined inflammatory processes. In particular, this chapter describes the modulatory role of the simplest forms of opioid peptides, Met-enkephalin and Leu-enkephalin, in antigen-associated inflammatory responses such as systemic and passive anaphylactic reactions, Arthus and delayed skin- hypersensitivity reactions, experimental allergic encephalomyelitis, allograft rejection, and adjuvant arthritis. For these studies, several schedules and various doses of enkephalins were employed in different immunoinflammatory paradigms. Bearing in mind that exogenous enkephalins are relatively rapidly degraded after in vivo administration (Roda et al. 1986), in the authors' study animals were repeatedly injected with pharmacological doses of enkephalins ranging from 10 mg/kg b.w. to 1 ng/kg b.w. After empirical definition of dose-dependent effects, the injection of a relatively high dose (5 mg/kg b.w.) had an opposite effect from that of a relatively low dose (0.2 mg/kg b.w.) of enkephalins. These modulatory activities were found to be reproducible. There was suppression with high and potentiation with low doses. Each type of immunoinflammatory reaction is dealt with separately.

Anaphylactic Reaction

Anaphylaxis (Portier and Richet 1902) is an inflammatory reaction of the immediate hypersensitivity type which occurs after reexposure of a sensitized animal to a corresponding antigen. The section concerns anaphylactic shock, passive cutaneous anaphylaxis, mast cell degranulation, and IgE production in relation to enkephalins.

In the rat, histamine and serotonin have been shown directly to mediate systemic anaphylactic reactions (Sanyal and West 1958). However, recent in vitro and in vivo studies suggest that the expression of immediate hypersensitivity reactions can also be modulated by neuropeptides such as somatostatin (Payan et al. 1984; Goetzl et al. 1985), substance P (Hagermark et al. 1978; Foreman and Jordan 1983), neurotensin (Foreman et al. 1982), vasoactive intestinal peptide

(Morice et al. 1983), dynorphin and β-endorphin (Casale et al. 1984; Bernton et al. 1985), and thyrotropin-releasing hormone (Bernton et al. 1985). As to the role of opioids in different types of shock (endotoxic, hemorrhagic, spinal and anaphylactic), since the level of β-endorphin was increased, it was suggested that this 31 amino acid neuropeptide exerts a direct influence on the pathogenesis of shock (Guillemin et al. 1977; Carr et al. 1982; Oyama et al. 1983). Furthermore, it has been anticipated that β-endorphin stimulates mast cell degranulation and histamine release through specific opioid receptors (Casale et al. 1984) and thus exacerbates the shock and increases the mortality rate. On the other hand, γ-endorphin (16 amino acid N-terminal fragment of β-endorphin) and its non-opioid analogue Des-Tyr-γ-endorphin exert a beneficial effect in anaphylactic shock by antagonizing the effect of β-endorphin (Amir and Ree 1985). Furthermore, the mast cell membrane possesses receptors for dynorphin (κ agonist) and D-Ala^2-D-Leu^5-enkephalin (δ agonist), and these receptors have also been implicated in the modulation of histamine release by mast cells (Casale et al. 1984). Thus, it seems that different opioid peptides play distinct roles in anaphylactic shock.

A detailed in vivo study on the relationship between enkephalin and anaphylactic shock in the rat (Janković and Marić 1987b) was carried out as follows. Wistar rats, sensitized for systemic anaphylaxis with subcutaneous injections of crystalline ovalbumin in aluminum hydroxide gel, received ten intraperitoneal injections containing a pharmacologically high dose (5 mg/kg b.w.) of Met-enkephalin or Leu-enkephalin, 5 days before the induction of anaphylactic shock. Thirty minutes after the last injection of enkephalin or saline (in the control group) each animal was challenged intravenously with a shocking dose of ovalbumin. The occurrence of anaphylactic symptoms, severity of clinical signs, and mortality rate were recorded for each group of rats. From serum samples obtained 12 h before the challenge for anaphylactic shock, the IgE levels were determined by passive cutaneous anaphylaxis, enzyme-linked immunosorbent assay, and paper radio-allergosorbent test and IgG antibody by use of a passive microhemagglutination method. Mast cell degranulation in the omentum was examined in each animal at autopsy.

Both enkephalins, Met-enkephalin in particular, significantly inhibited the development of systemic anaphylaxis in the rat (Table 1). The most important finding was that ten injections of Met-enkephalin completely protect the animals from fatal shock. In these animals IgE level and percentage of degranulated mast cells were very low. These observations seem to imply that Met-enkephalin is a potent anti-anaphylactic agent which can be employed in the prevention of anaphylactic shock and related immune reactions (Table 1). Met-enkephalin and Leu-enkephalin also decrease the production of circulating anti-albumin IgE and IgG antibodies and mast cell degranulation. Thus, it seems that native enkephalins, and particularly Met-enkephalin, can modulate the inflammatory reaction of the anaphylactic type by decreasing the synthesis and/or release of antigen-specific homocytotropic antibodies and thus the sensitization of mast cells.

Table 1. Anaphylactic reaction in rats sensitized with ovalbumin, treated with high (5 mg/kg) dose of methionine-enkephalin (Met-Enk) or leucine-enkephalin (Leu-Enk), and intravenously challenged with a shock dose of ovalbumin

Treatment	Intensity of clinical signs of anaphylactic shock (mean score)	Total mortality rate (%)	Circulatory IgE titer			Circulatory IgG titer (log_2)	Degranulated mast cells at autopsy (%)
			PCA titer (log_2)	ELISA titer (log_2)	PRAST (U/ml)		
Saline	3.1 ± 0.5	75	4.3 ± 0.5	8.0 ± 0.7	7.6 ± 3.5	6.9 ± 0.6	78.1 ± 5.8
Met-Enk	$0.9 \pm 0.7^{a,b}$	0	$0.4 \pm 0.6^{a,b}$	$1.6 \pm 0.7^{a,b}$	$1.7 \pm 1.4^{a,b}$	$2.8 \pm 0.7^{a,b}$	$17.9 \pm 4.4^{a,b}$
Leu-Enk	2.0 ± 0.5^{a}	43	2.5 ± 0.5^{a}	5.5 ± 0.8^{a}	5.9 ± 2.1	4.6 ± 0.6^{a}	52.3 ± 6.6^{a}

Mean score, an arithmetic score reflecting overall intensity of reaction. PCA, passive cutaneous anaphylaxis; ELISA, enzyme-linked immonosorbent assay; PRAST, paper radio-allergosorbent test. Statistical significance determined by Student's *t* test; $^{a}p < 0.001$, enkephalin-treated group vs. saline-treated group; $^{b}p < 0.001$, Met-Enk-treated group vs Leu-Enk-treated group.

Since previous studies demonstrated that the production of antibodies to both particulate and soluble antigens is markedly diminished by a large dose of Met-enkephalin (Janković and Marić 1986, 1987a), and since this influence can be significantly prevented by antagonists specific for δ opioid receptors (Marić and Janković 1987b; Janković and Marić 1988), one may deduce that modulation of anaphylactic function by Met-enkephalin is, at least to a certain extent, mediated via δ receptors. In substantial agreement with this hypothesis are observations that enkephalins may impair B-lymphocyte function and thus produce abnormalities in antigen-specific antibody synthesis (Johnson et al. 1982), and that enkephalins can directly bind to δ-opioid receptors on mast cells and thus regulate degranulation of these cells (Casale et al. 1984). However, the involvement of other opioid and nonopioid receptors can not be excluded.

In addition, the suppression of anaphylactic shock induced by high doses of enkephalins should not be associated exclusively with the level of IgE and mast-cell damage and consequent release of monoamines. Still another possibility is that opioid peptides may contribute to the pathophysiology of the shock by their action on the central nervous system (CNS) and/or parasympathetic outflow and sympathetic tone (Holaday 1983). It is also possible that the mechanisms underlying anaphylactic shock are associated with the interaction of endorphins with enkephalins. As mentioned earlier, Amir and Ree (1985) described the relationship between γ-endorphin and β-endorphin, and suggested that γ- endorphin-type peptides exert antianaphylactic action by physiologically antagonizing the "autonomic" effects of β-endorphin, which exacerbates the shock. Concerning the enkephalins, since high doses of these peptides produce a beneficial effect in animals challenged with antigen one may assume that enkephalins act as potent modulators of β-endorphin action at the mast cell level, namely binding of enkephalin to δ-receptors prevents simultaneous binding of β-endorphin, the release of which is caused by the shock dose of antigen and thus inhibits mast cell degranulation and release of histamine. In the rat, however, anaphylactic shock is also characterized by an increase in the release of serotonin (Sanyal and West 1958). Therefore, enkephalin may interfere in anaphylactic shock by the release and action of serotonin.

Arthus Skin Reaction

The cutaneous Arthus Reaction (Arthus 1903) is a severe immediate inflammatory response to the injection of specific antigen into the skin of sensitized animals. Biochemically, immune complexes activate the complement system and act on platelets and mast cells to release vasoactive amines (Humphrey and Jaques 1954; Barbero 1961), increasing blood flow and capillary permeability and consequent migration of PMN from blood vessels into the tissues (Jensen et al. 1969; Ward 1969).

Table 2. Arthus skin hypersensitivity reaction in rats sensitized with BSA, treated with high or low doses of methionine-enkephalin (Met-Enk) or leucine-enkephalin (Leu-Enk), and skin tested with BSA

Treatment	Dose (mg/kg)	Anti-BSA antibody titer ($\log_2$)	Arthus reaction		
			Diameter of reaction (mm)	Severity of reaction (mean score)	Positive reaction (%)
Saline		7.2 ± 0.5	13.0 ± 2.5	1.8 ± 0.6	100
Met-Enk	5	$2.8 \pm 0.6^{a,b,d}$	$6.1 \pm 3.0^{a,b,d}$	$0.4 \pm 0.5^{a,b}$	25
	0.2	$9.5 \pm 0.6^{a,e}$	$24.4 \pm 3.6^{a,e}$	2.8 ± 0.5^{a}	100
Leu-Enk	5	$5.5 \pm 0.5^{a,c}$	$9.2 \pm 2.1^{a,c}$	$0.7 \pm 0.7^{a,c}$	38
	0.2	8.7 ± 0.5^{a}	19.3 ± 3.2^{a}	2.5 ± 0.4^{a}	100

Statistical significance determined by Student's t test: $^{a}p < 0.001$, enkephalin-treated group vs. saline-treated group; $^{b}p < 0.001$, high dose of Met-Enk vs. low dose of Met-Enk; $^{c}p < 0.001$, high dose of Leu-Enk vs. low dose of Leu-Enk; $^{d}p < 0.001$, high dose of Met-Enk vs. high dose of Leu-Enk; $^{e}p < 0.001$, low dose of Met-Enk vs. low dose of Leu-Enk.

Studies with enkephalin have shown that these pentapeptides exert both inflammation-stimulating and inflammation-depressing properties (Janković and Marić 1986, 1987a; Marić and Janković 1987a). Wistar rats sensitized with bovine serum albumin (BSA) in complete Freund's adjuvant and treated daily for a period of 2 weeks with intraperitoneal injections containing pharmacologically high (5 mg/kg b.w.) or low (0.2 mg/kg b.w.) doses of enkephalin and then skin tested with BSA exhibited dose-dependent Arthus reactions. High doses of enkephalin, Met-enkephalin in particular, markedly suppressed both the incidence and intensity of the Arthus reaction (Table 2) whereas low doses of these pentapeptides potentiated the reaction.

Direct correlation of intensity of Arthus reactions with anti-BSA titers after administration of high and low doses of enkephalins implies that these pentapeptides exert their effect on the Arthus reaction by modulating the release of specific antibody. Indeed, antibody synthesis depends on the dose of enkephalin (Gungor et al. 1980; Johnson et al. 1982; Heijnen et al. 1986; Janković and Marić 1986, 1987a). In addition, histological analysis of the reaction revealed in saline-treated control animals an appreciable infiltration of PMN located at or near the small blood vessels. However, pretreatment of animals with high doses of enkephalin produced a striking depletion of PMN. On the other hand, low doses of these opioids increased the number of PMN. These findings imply that enkephalins may also exert their activity via reaction with nonspecific inflammatory effector cells. Indeed, it has been reported (Simkins et al. 1984; Ruff et al. 1985) that enkephalins may act either in a stimulatory or an inhibitory manner on the chemotactic activity of PMN and thus affect the migration of these cells toward inflammatory foci. This interaction of opioids with PMN is most probably mediated specifically through opioid receptors (Falke and Fischer

1985; Stefano, this volume). However, the involvement of platelets (Mehrishi and Mills 1983) and vascular endothelial cells (Boogaerts et al. 1983) may also play an active role in the development of Arthus reactivity due to the presence of receptors for opioid peptides on these cells.

Delayed Hypersensitivity Skin Reaction

The delayed hypersensitivity skin reaction is an immunologically determined local inflammatory response characterized by relatively slow development (within 72 h) following intradermal injection of antigen into an appropriately sensitized animal (Vassalli and McCluskey 1971). Histologically, the common feature is the presence of $CD4^+$ lymphocytes, then macrophages, PMN, and Langerhans cells. Biochemically, there are production and release of soluble mediators, collectively termed cytokines, which produce a variety of biological activities from the recruitment to the activation of lymphocytes, macrophages, PMN, and other inflmmatory cells at the site of the lesion (Wells 1984).

The delayed-type of skin-hypersensitivity reaction to purified BSA in rats was studied (Marić and Janković 1987a). Animals were sensitized to BSA by a single inoculation of 0.5 mg BSA in complete Freund's adjuvant into a footpad, and delayed hypersensitivity reaction was induced 14 days later by an intradermal injection of 30 μg BSA in 0.1 ml saline. The inflammatory response was recorded at 24 h. Grossly, the inflammatory reaction was evaluated by mean diameter (mm), and degree of induration graded on an arbitrary scale (0 to + + + +). Microscopic examination of the site of reaction revealed characteristic infiltrations of lymphocytes and macrophages.

Treatment of sensitized animals with intraperitoneal injections containing high (5 mg/kg b.w.) and low (0.2 mg/kg b.w.) doses of enkephalin, administered for 14 consecutive days after immunization, produced dose-dependent effects on the delayed inflammatory response to BSA. High doses of enkephalin induced a striking decrease, both in incidence and intensity, of delayed reactions to BSA whereas low doses produced significant potentiation of these reactions (Table 3). Histologically, in rats given high doses of enkephalin skin reactions showed a marked depletion of mononuclear cells. By contrast, low doses of pentapeptides increased the number of inflammatory cells in comparison with saline-treated control animals.

As to the mechanism(s) of enkephalin-induced modulation of delayed-type inflammatory responses, one possibility is that these peptides act on antigen-specific T-lymphocytes. Several in vitro assays suggest that opioid peptides may induce potentiation and suppression of antigen/mitogen-induced T-cell blastogenesis and proliferation (Puppo et al. 1985; Barabino et al. 1986; McCain et al. 1986; Plotnikoff et al. 1986). Furthermore, Met-enkephalin and other opioid peptides have been shown to suppress $CD8^+$ cells and to release T-lymphocyte chemotactic factor (Brown and Van Epps 1985), which may play an important

Table 3. Delayed hypersensitivity skin reaction in rats sensitized with BSA, treated with high or low doses of methionine-enkephalin (Met-Enk) or leucine-enkephalin (Leu-Enk), and skin tested with BSA

Treatment	Dose (mg/kg)	Delayed reaction		
		Mean diameter of reaction (%)	Severity of reaction (mean score)	Positive reaction (%)
Saline		15.2 ± 2.0	2.6 ± 0.5	100
Met-Enk	5	$7.7 \pm 2.6^{a,b,d}$	$0.6 \pm 0.6^{a,b,d}$	56
	0.2	$25.1 \pm 3.1^{a,e}$	$3.9 \pm 0.6^{a,e}$	100
Leu-Enk	5	$11.0 \pm 2.2^{a,c}$	$1.3 \pm 0.4^{a,c}$	63
	0.2	19.7 ± 3.0^{a}	3.2 ± 0.5^{a}	100

Mean score, an arithmetic score reflecting overall intensity of reaction. Statistical significance determined by Student's t test: $^{a}p < 0.001$, enkephalin-treated group vs. saline-treated group; $^{b}p < 0.001$, high dose of Met-Enk vs. low dose of Met-Enk; $^{c}p < 0.001$, high dose of Leu-Enk vs. low dose of Leu-Enk; $^{d}p < 0.001$, high dose of Met-Enk vs. high dose of Leu-Enk; $^{e}p < 0.001$, low dose of Met-Enk vs. low dose of Leu-Enk.

role in inflammatory processes of the delayed type by specifically attracting $CD4^{+}$ cells to inflammatory foci (Van Epps et al. 1983). In addition, opioid peptides, and Met-enkephalin in particular, may act directly as lymphocytotactic factors by binding to the opioid peptide-specific receptors present on lymphocytes (Van Epps and Saland 1984). Enkephalins may also exert their immunomodulatory function via opioid receptors of nonspecific inflammatory cells which take part in delayed hypersensitivity skin reactions. For example, these peptides have been shown to upregulate or downregulate macrophage-effector functions such as cytotoxicity and phagocytosis (Foris et al. 1986), and superoxide production (Sharp et al. 1985). The action of opioid peptides on inflammation-related mediators released at sites remote from the inflammatory reactions should also be taken into consideration.

Experimental Allergic Encephalomyelitis

Experimental allergic encephalomyelitis (EAE) is an autoimmune, inflammatory, demyelinating disease of the CNS (Kabat et al. 1947) which occurs after immunization with homologous or heterologous CNS tissue, myelin basic protein (MBP), or certain polypeptide sequences of MBP (Kies and Alvord 1959; Paterson 1960; Orgad and Cohen 1974; Hashim 1978; Hashim et al. 1978).

Since T-lymphocytes are the crucial inflammatory cells in EAE (Hickey et al. 1983; Traugott 1985), and the function of these cells can be affected by different mediators (Paterson et al. 1981), we hypothesized that manipulation of EAE with opioid pentapeptides may modulate this autoimmune disease (Janković and Marić 1987c). Lewis rats were challenged with fresh guinea pig spinal cord in complete Freund's adjuvant, inoculated into a hindfoot pad, and then treated for a period of 17 consecutive days with intraperitoneal injections containing either a high dose (5 mg/kg b.w.) or a low dose (0.2 mg/kg b.w.) of Met-enkephalin or Leu-enkephalin. EAE in these animals was assessed by severity of clinical signs and histological lesions in the CNS.

The high dose of Met-enkephalin significantly delayed the onset of EAE and markedly inhibited the neurological signs of the disease and the development of mononuclear lesions in the CNS (Table 4). The loss of body weight which accompanies EAE was also prevented by a high dose of Met-enkephalin. By contrast, the low dose of this pentapeptide potentiated neurological and histopathological features of the disease compared to saline-treated sensitized controls. Leu-enkephalin failed to modulate EAE.

Furthermore, the high dose of Met-enkephalin successfully suppressed the adaptive transfer of EAE in the rat (Janković and Marić 1990) namely, lymphocytes from donors sensitized with encephalitogen and treated for 10 days with a 5 mg/kg b.w. dose of Met-enkephalin were unable to transfer the disease to nonimmunized saline-treated recipients or to recipients which received daily injections of a 5 mg/kg dose of Met-enkephalin over a period of 7 consecutive days after the transfer of cells (Table 5). Similarly, lymphocytes from sensitized saline-treated donors failed to transfer EAE to nonsensitized Met-enkephalin treated recipients. The disease was successfully transferred only when lymphocytes from sensitized saline-treated donors were inoculated into normal saline-treated recipients. These recipients, 7 days after cell transfer, developed CNS lesions characteristic of EAE. Results of the transfer study suggest that Met-enkephalin inhibits the capacity of lymphoid cells from normal donors sensitized with encephalitogen to convey the disease, and the ability of Met-enkephalin treated recipients to accept EAE-reactive cells from saline-treated donors. It seems, therefore, that this opioid peptide affects both the function of EAE effector cells in donors and the properties of the recipient microenvironment necessary for the expression of transferred EAE effector lymphocytes.

Although the available experimental and clinical evidence does not permit a complete understanding of the EAE-immunoregulatory network in which enkephalins are involved, it does suggest the following modulation of specific encephalitic receptor activity on T-lymphocytes: (a) Met-enkephalin binds to lymphocyte receptors reactive in EAE and thus modulates or blocks their function; (b) Met-enkephalin acts directly on effector T-lymphocytes and modifies their specificity and reactivity to encephalitogenic molecules situated on the suface of neurons; and (c) if receptors on the lymphocyte membrane are located in close vicinity to opioid receptors, Met-enkephalin binding may be involved in the EAE process. The possibility of interaction of Met-enkephalin with the encephalitogen-specific B-lymphocyte, which regulates important humoral immune reactions in EAE (Janković et al. 1965; Gausas et al. 1982), cannot be

Table 4. Development of EAE in rats sensitized with guinea pig spinal cord and treated with high or low doses of methionine-enkephalin (Met-Enk) or leucine-enkephalin (Leu-Enk)

Treatment	Dose (mg/kg)	Average day of onset of EAE	Intensity of clinical signs of EAE (mean score)	Percentage of rats with EAE paralysis	Intensity of histopathological signs of EAE (mean score)	Percentage of rats with EAE histopathological lesions
Saline		13.0 ± 0.1	2.5 ± 0.1	70.0 ± 4.9	2.8 ± 0.2	95.4 ± 8.1
Met-Enk	5	$16.5 \pm 0.2^{a,b,c}$	$0.6 \pm 0.2^{a,b,c}$	$10.8 \pm 5.6^{a,b,c}$	$0.9 \pm 0.1^{a,b,c}$	$41.3 \pm 9.6^{a,b,c}$
	0.2	$10.0 \pm 0.1^{a,d}$	$3.8 \pm 0.2^{a,d}$	$83.4 \pm 7.3^{a,d}$	$3.9 \pm 0.2^{a,d}$	100
Leu-Enk	5	13.1 ± 0.1	2.4 ± 0.2	68.4 ± 7.8	2.9 ± 0.2	90.8 ± 14.3
	0.2	13.3 ± 0.2	2.4 ± 0.2	69.1 ± 6.2	3.0 ± 0.2	93.3 ± 10.2

Mean scores, arithmetic scores reflecting overall intensity of clinical/histopathology. Statistical significance determined by Student's t test: $^{a}p < 0.001$, enkephalin-treated group vs. saline-treated group; $^{b}p < 0.001$, high dose of Met-Enk vs. low dose of Met-Enk; $^{c}p < 0.001$, high dose of Met-Enk vs. high dose of Leu-Enk; $^{d}p < 0.001$, low dose of Met-Enk vs. low dose of Leu-Enk.

Table 5. The effect of high (5 mg/kg) dose of methionine-enkephalin (Met-Enk) on adaptive transfer of experimental allergic encephalomyelitis

Donors and recipients	Treatment	*n*	Mean histopathological lesions (no. of rats)					Mean score	Percentage of rats with lesions
			0	+	++	+++	++++		
Group A									
Donors	Saline	32	5	4	13	10	0	1.9 ± 0.2^{a}	84.4 ± 8.7^{a}
Recipients	Saline	12	0	0	1	7	4	3.2 ± 0.2^{b}	100
	Met-Enk	12	11	1	0	0	0	0.1 ± 0.1	8.3 ± 6.2
Group B									
Donors	Met-Enk	46	22	23	1	0	0	0.5 ± 0.1	52.2 ± 7.0
Recipients	Saline	14	12	2	0	0	0	0.1 ± 0.1	14.3 ± 8.3
	Met-Enk	13	12	1	0	0	0	0.1 ± 0.1	7.7 ± 6.4

Donors received ten daily injections of saline or Met-Enk (5 mg/kg b.w.); recipients received daily injections of saline or Met-Enk (5 mg/kg b.w.). An arithmetic mean score reflecting overall histological changes was calculated for each group of rats depending on the degree of lesions, defined as follows: 0 = 0; + = 1; ++ = 2; +++ = 3; and ++++ = 4. Negative animals are included in the calculation of means. Statistical significance determined by Student's *t* test: $^{a}p < 0.001$, saline-treated donors vs. Met-Enk-treated donors; $^{b}p < 0.001$, saline-treated recipients vs. Met-Enk-treated recipients.

excluded. Although in this study of EAE and enkephalin anti-brain antibody production was not measured, earlier experiments on nonnervous tissue antibody formation showed that high doses of these peptides suppress whereas low doses potentiate humoral immune responses in vivo (Janković and Marić 1986, 1987a). Thus, by analogy, Met-enkephalin may affect the development of EAE by modulating antibodies specific for nervous tissue antigens. Finally, enkephalin may be operating through nonspecific inflammatory cells such as macrophages, monocytes, endothelial cells, or astrocytes.

For almost five decades EAE has been extensively studied as an animal model for human demyelinating diseases, and a variety of substances and treatments have been tested in an effort to ameliorate the clinical and histopathological signs of the disease. The pronounced immunousuppressing effect of Met-enkephalin on EAE in the rat, as described here, raises the possibility that this opioid peptide might be used in the treatment of inflammatory demyelinating diseases in animals and humans. Indeed, in a preliminary study Marić and Janković (1988) described the therapeutic effect of Met-enkephalin on EAE in Lewis rats immunized with encephalitogen. Once the first EAE symptom (e.g., flaccid tail) occurred, the animals were treated intraperitoneally with 5 mg/kg b.w. of Met-enkephalin every 12 h for 7 consecutive days. Immunized controls were given saline injections. Rats were carefully inspected for clinical signs of EAE, killed at the end of the treatment, and CNS tissues processed for histological examination. Saline-treated rats developed within 7 days severe EAE paralysis and pronounced mononuclear inflammatory lesions in the cerebrum, cerebellum, and spinal cord. By contrast, several rats given Met-enkephalin completely recovered from the disease; there was no progression of clinical signs, and histopathological lesions in the CNS were rare and mild.

Pertinent to the possible therapeutic effect of Met-enkephalin is a recent study with three patients suffering from severe progressive multiple sclerosis. They were given intrathecal injections of Met-enkephalin, and none of these patients showed progression of the disease for a period of 3 years of clinical observation (Janković et al. 1989a).

Allograft Rejection

The phenomenon of graft rejection between unrelated individuals is another example of delayed inflammatory immune response in which the contact of the donor's alloantigens with the host's immunocytes results in severe inflammatory destruction of grafted cells. Since allograft rejection is mediated by antigen-specific and nonspecific inflammatory cells and involves a variety of humoral factors, many of them mentioned in the preceding sections, it was logical to assume that opioid pentapeptides may also take part in inflammatory processes underlying allograft rejection. Therefore, the effect of enkephalin on the survival rate of a thyroid allograft implanted under the kidney capsule was investigated.

For this purpose, thyroid tissue from a Lewis donor rat was surgically implanted under the capsule of the right kidney of a Wistar recipient. Thereafter, recipients were given intraperitoneally 5 mg/kg b.w. of Met-enkephalin or Leu-enkephalin every 12 h for a period of 4 consecutive days. Control recipients were treated with saline in the same manner. Kidney grafts were removed 5 days after transplantation, and processed for histological appraisal. Allograft rejection was determined microscopically by the degree of infiltration of the thyroid parenchyma with the host's mononuclear cells and graded on an arbitrary scale.

Enkephalin significantly prolonged the survival of the thyroid allograft; Met-enkephalin was much more effective in delaying allograft rejection than Leu-enkephalin (Table 6). Histologically, the thyroid graft of enkephalin-treated recipients showed a large number of well-preserved follicles, and weak interstitial infiltration of host mononuclear cells covering about 5%–10% of the graft tissue. By contrast, the thyroid implants of saline-treated control recipients exhibited almost complete destruction of follicles and extensive infiltration (up to 80%) of the graft parenchyma with invading mononuclear host cells.

These results suggest that enkephalins, Met-enkephalin in particular, exert a potent anti-inflammatory effect on inflammatory processes of allograft rejection. As to the mechanisms by which enkephalins prolong the survival of the allograft, they may be similar to enkephalin effects described in the previous sections. Three possibilities, not mutually exclusive, are mentioned here. First, enkephalin may act directly on antigen-specific $CD4^+$ lymphocytes and thus postpone the initial phase of inflammatory reaction. Second, this pentapeptide may "suppress" the production of $CD8^+$ T-suppressor lymphocytes by a T-lymphocyte chemotactic factor which attracts $CD4^+$ cells to the inflammatory foci (Van Epps et al. 1983). Third, enkephalin may diminish the antigen-specific cytotoxic capacity of T-cells (Prete et al. 1986) and thus the survival of the allograft.

The peptides can also influence the function of other inflammatory cells, such as NK cells (Wybran 1985; Prete et al. 1986) and macrophages (Foris et al. 1986). Binding of enkephalin to specific opioid peptide receptors present on the

Table 6. Rejection of allogenic thyroid graft implanted under the kidney capsule of rats treated with high (5 mg/kg) dose of methionine-enkephalin (Met-Enk) or leucine-enkephalin (Leu-Enk)

Treatment	n	Degree of rejection on day 5 after implantation					Mean score
		0	+	++	+++	++++	
Saline	24	0	0	0	8	16	3.7 ± 0.5
Met-Enk	20	6	14	0	0	0	$0.7 \pm 0.5^{a,c}$
Leu-Enk	20	0	3	16	1	0	1.9 ± 0.4^{b}

Results are expressed in terms of a histological evaluation of rejection. Mean score, an arithmetic score reflecting an overall intensity of reaction defined as follows: 0 = 0; + = 1; + + = 2; + + + = 3; and + + + + = 4. Statistical significance determined by Student's t test: $^{a}p < 0.001$, Met-Enk-treated group vs. saline-treated group; $^{b}p < 0.001$, Leu-Enk-treated group vs. saline-treated group; $^{c}p < 0.001$, Met-Enk-treated group vs. Leu-Enk-treated group.

membranes of these cells (Mathews et al. 1983; Foris et al. 1984; Scharrer and Stefano, this volume) can modulate their functional (Koff and Dunegan 1985; Sharp et al. 1985), cytotoxic (Foris et al. 1984; Mandler et al. 1986), and chemotactic (Ruff et al. 1985) activities in allograft rejection. Although the precise mechanism of enkephalin-induced modulation of host-graft reactions cannot yet be defined, the antiallograft rejection activity of enkephalin, as described here, suggests the possible use of these opioid pentapeptides, particularly of Met-enkephalin, in clinical practice.

Adjuvant Arthritis

Adjuvant arthritis is an experimentally induced immunelike inflammatory disorder in which laboratory animals develop polyarthritis 8–14 days after a single inoculation with complete Freund's adjuvant into one footpad (Pearson 1956; Pearson and Wood 1959).

Because opioid pentapeptides are known to modulate inflammatory reactions in vivo, an attempt was made to manipulate the development of adjuvant arthritis by administration of high and low doses of Met-enkephalin and Leu-enkephalin. Wistar rats were inoculated in one hind footpad with 0.3 ml of complete Freund's adjuvant, and then injected intraperitoneally every 24 h with 5 mg/kg or 0.2 mg/kg of enkephalin for a period of 14 consecutive days. The appearance and severity of adjuvant arthritis was ascertained by comparing inflammatory enlargements of the adjuvant-injected and the contralateral noninjected foot, the appearance of cutaneous and subcutaneous nodules in the tail, perivascular lesions in the external ear, and increased weights of ipsilateral and contralateral inguinal lymph nodes. The high dose of Met-enkephalin produced a striking decrease of the inflammatory reaction of joints and lymph nodes of the leg inoculated with adjuvant (Table 7). On the other hand, the high dose of Leu-enkephalin produced only a mild anti-inflammatory effect on the adjuvant-injected foot and regional lymph nodes. Inflammatory reactions in the ears were also less pronounced in animals treated with high doses of enkephalin compared to saline-treated controls. In contrast, the low dose of Met-enkephalin enhanced the inflammatory reactions characteristic of adjuvant arthritis.

Histopathologically, in saline-treated rats there was an extensive disruption of the basic cellular makeup of the ipsilateral inguinal lymph nodes induced by the complete Freund's adjuvant. There was partial or complete replacement of primary and secondary lymphoid nodules and germinal centers, and paracortical lymphocytes by inflammatory cells and proliferating connective tissue. However, in animals given the high dose of Met-enkephalin the cellular architecture of the regional lymph nodes was less affected.

The results of this study imply that enkephalins, and Met-enkephalin in particular, may act as physiological modulators of inflammatory processes related to adjuvant arthritis. Since T-lymphocytes probably play a regulatory

Table 7. Development of adjuvant arthritis in rats sensitized with complete Freund's adjuvant and treated with high or low doses of methionine-enkephalin (Met-Enk) or leucine-enkephalin (Leu-Enk)

Treatment	Dose (mg/kg)	Diameter of the foot (mm)			Weight of inguinal lymph nodes (μg/g b.w.)		
		Injected foot	Noninjected foot	Difference	Injected foot	Noninjected foot	Difference
Saline		12.8 ± 3.2	5.0 ± 0.4	7.8 ± 2.3	419.4 ± 73.2	61.4 ± 13.2	358.0 ± 62.1
Met-Enk	5	7.8 ± 2.5[a,b]	4.9 ± 0.7	2.9 ± 1.8[a,b]	201.8 ± 42.7[a,b,d]	58.1 ± 12.7	143.7 ± 30.9[a,b,d]
	0.2	17.7 ± 3.0[a,e]	5.1 ± 0.6	12.6 ± 2.6[a,e]	523.0 ± 52.6[a,e]	54.3 ± 12.1	468.7 ± 36.7[a,e]
Leu-Enk	5	10.0 ± 1.9[c]	5.7 ± 0.6	4.3 ± 2.0[a,c]	336.5 ± 80.3[a,c]	63.2 ± 13.7	273.3 ± 69.8[a,c]
	0.2	13.6 ± 3.1	6.6 ± 0.8	7.0 ± 2.1	418.5 ± 61.2	57.6 ± 11.9	360.9 ± 48.3

Statistical significance determined by Student's t test: [a]$p < 0.001$, enkephalin-treated group vs. saline-treated group; [b]$p < 0.001$, high dose of Met-Enk vs. low dose of Met-Enk; [c]$p < 0.001$, high dose of Leu-Enk vs. low dose of Leu-Enk; [d]$p < 0.001$, high dose of Met-Enk vs. high dose of Leu-Enk; [e]$p < 0.001$, low dose of Met-Enk vs. low dose of Leu-Enk.

role in adjuvant arthritis (Kayashima et al. 1976), and since these cells can bind enkephalin through specific opioid receptors, one may deduce that in adjuvant arthritis there is a direct and specific interaction of these pentapeptides with antigen-reactive T-cells. However, interactions of enkephalin with other antigen-specific or nonspecific inflammatory cells in adjuvant arthritis cannot be excluded. No matter which mechanism may prove to be effective, the potent anti-inflammatory activity of Met-enkephalin in adjuvant arthritis should stimulate clinical trials with this drug in rheumatoid and other inflammatory arthritic disorders in humans.

Concluding Remarks

Various pharmacological, immunological, histochemical, and biochemical methods have demonstrated that opioid peptides and their specific receptors play an important role in the regulation of a variety of physiological processes in the organism. However, the influence of opioid peptides on lymphocytes and immune responses has received attention only very recently. Both opioid and nonopioid receptors were detected on immunocompetent cells, and these cells were found to synthesize and secrete opioid peptide precursors and fragments. Thus far, the great majority of immunological studies have attempted to elucidate opioid peptide activity by testing one particular peptide in vitro. By contrast, the authors' results referred to are based on an in vivo strategy. This chapter provides evidence for the immunomodulating activity of two opioid pentapeptides, Met-enkephalin and Leu-enkephalin, on various immunoinflammatory responses in the rat, i.e., systemic anaphylaxis, Arthus and delayed-hypersensitivity skin reactions, experimental allergic encephalomyelitis, allograft rejection, and adjuvant arthritis.

Apparently the enkephalins exert a dual, dose-dependent activity, i.e., large doses suppress whereas small doses enhance different inflammatory immune paradigms. Met-enkephalin and Leu-enkephalin differ only in C-terminal amino acid; their immunomodulating activities do not. Met-enkephalin is generally more effective than Leu-enkephalin. This difference may be related to their preference for different opioid receptors μ, δ, and κ (see also Stefano, this volume). Met-enkephalin interacts primarily with δ-receptors and shows a somewhat reduced but still significant affinity for μ-receptors (Paterson et al. 1984). On the other hand, Leu-enkephalin binds primarily but not exclusively to μ receptors. These distinctions are in substantial agreement with the observations (Marić and Janković 1987b) that the immunomodulatory activity of Met-enkephalin, but not that of Leu-enkephalin, is strikingly reduced in the presence of ICI 174864, a specific antagonist for δ receptors whereas naloxone used in small doses reacts primarily with μ opioid receptors (Janković and Marić 1988).

The question arises as to whether the affinity of enkephalins for respective receptors depends on their conformational states. Given the nature of this conformation-dependent phenomenon, it surely does. Conformational energy calculations of the zwitterionic form of Met-enkephalin suggested that about 15 different extended or folded forms of this peptide may be found in solution (De Cohen et al. 1977). On the other hand, an X-ray structural study revealed the existence of four distinct independent Leu-enkephalin molecules, each one of different extended conformation (Smith and Griffin 1978). It has been assumed that folded structures of enkephalin may preferentially interact with the μ receptor, whereas the extended forms prefer the δ receptor (Schiller 1984). Thus, the differences between immunomodulatory effects of Met-enkephalin and Leu-enkephalin in various inflammatory reactions, as described here, may be due to different conformational states of these pentapeptides in a given micro-environment and to variations in the binding activity of these opioids to distinct classes of opioid receptors. The occurrence of different types of conformational structures of Met-enkephalin and Leu-enkephalin indicates the flexibility of the enkephalin molecules and dependence of their conformation on microenvironmental factors. This property may be of great importance for the involvement of enkephalin in a variety of biochemical processes in the organism, including those related to the immune system.

The difference in the activity of the two peptides may also be ascribed to the time required for their inactivation by endogenous enzymes (Hambrook et al. 1976; see Turner et al., this volume). Recent developments have shown, however, that plasma components may act as carriers for enkephalins and thus protect them from enzyme hydrolysis (Possenti et al. 1983). Since these protecting mechanisms may be unequally efficient, the half-lives of two enkephalins under in vivo conditions may also be different (Roda et al. 1986). Moreover, the immunomodulation-related discrepancy between Met-enkephalin and Leu-enkephalin may be attributed to differences between enkephalins in gaining access to the interior of the cells by a process of internalization protecting them from peptidases. The process of internalization may occur in lymphocytes as well as other inflammation-associated cells. However, this possibility has yet to be evaluated experimentally. Finally, one may hypothesize that competition between inoculated enkephalin and endogenous enkephalin produced by lymphocytes and other cells (Smith et al. 1985) constitutes a balance for in vivo immunomodulatory effects. Indeed, treatment of rats with exogenous Met-enkephalin induces changes at the level of endogenous opioid ligands, suggesting a relationship between exogenous and endogenous opioid ligands in immunomodulation (Janković et al. 1989b). The proposed biochemical interpretation of enkephalinergic immunoregulation is preliminary.

Acknowledgements. The authors' research referred to in this chapter was supported by the Republic of Serbia Research Fund, Belgrade, Yugoslavia.

References

Amir S, Ree JM (1985) Beneficial effect of γ-endorphin-type peptides in anaphylactic shock. Brain Res 329:329–333

Arthus M (1903) Injections répétées de serum de cheval chez le lapin. CR Soc Biol 55:817

Atweh SF, Kuhar MJ (1983) Distribution and physiological significance of opioid receptors in the brain. Br Med Bull 39:47–52

Barabino A, Morgano A, Pierri I, Rogna S, Lotti G, Indiveri F (1986) Effect of α-endorphin on mixed lymphocyte reaction in young and aged healty donors. Top Aging Res Eur 9:143–147

Barbero JF (1961) The release of histamine from rabbit platelets by means of antigen-antibody precipitates. I. The precipitation of the immune complex in histamine release. J Immunol 86:369–376

Beaumont A, Hughes J (1979) Biology of opioid peptides. Annu Rev Pharmacol Toxicol 19:245–267

Bernton EW, Long JB, Holaday JW (1985) Opioids and neuropeptides: mechanism in circulatory shock. Fed Proc 44:290–299

Bloom F, Segal D, Ling N, Guillemin R (1976) Endorphins: profound behavioral effects in rats suggest new etiological factors in mental illness. Science 194:630–632

Boogaerts MA, Vermylen J, Deckmyn H, Roelant C, Verwilghen RL, Jacob HS, Moldow CF (1983) Enkephalins modify granulocyte-endothelial cell interactions by stimulating prostacyclin production. Thromb haemost 50:572–576

Brown SL, Van Epps DE (1985) Suppression of T-lymphocyte chemotactic factor production by the opioid peptides beta-endorphin and Met-enkephalin. J Immunol 134:3384–3390

Carr DB, Bergland R, Hamilton A, Blume H, Kasting N, Arnold M, Martin JB, Rosenblatt M (1982) Endotoxin-stimulated opioid peptide secretion: two secretory pools and feedback control in vivo. Science 217:845–848

Car DJJ (1988) Opioid receptors on cells of the immune system. Prog-Neuroendocrinimmunol 1:8–14

Car DJJ, Klimpel GR (1986) Enhancement of the generation of cytotoxic T-cells by endogenous opiates. J Neuroimmunol 12:75–87

Casale JB, Bowman S, Kaliner M (1984) Induction of human cutaneous mast cell degranulation by opiates and endogenous opioid peptides. Evidence for opiate and nonopiate receptor participation. J Allergy Clin Immunol 73:775–781

Cohnheim J (1867) Über Entzündung und Eiterung. Arch Pathol Anat 40:1

Conroy MC, Adkinson NF, Lichtenstein LM (1977) Measurement of IgE on human basophils. Relation to serum lgE and anti-lgE induced histamine release. J Immunol 118:1317–1321

Cox BM, Opheim KE, Teschemacher H, Goldstein A (1975) A peptide- like substance from pituitary that acts like morphine. Life Sci 16:1777–1782

De Cohen JL, Humblat C, Koch MJH (1977) Theoretical conformational analysis of Met-enkephalin. FEBS Lett 73:38–42

Dobbins JW, Dharmsathaphrn K, Racusen L, Binder HJ (1981) The effect of somatostatin and enkephalin on ion transport in the intestine. Ann NY Acad Sci 372:594–612

Dvorak HF, Mihm MC, Dvorak AM, Johnson RA, Manseam EJ, Morgan E, Colvin RB (1974) Morphology of delayed type hypersensitivity reactions in man. I. Quantitative description of the inflammation response. Lab Invest 31:111–130

Enrich WE (1956) Die Entzündung. In: Buchner F, Letterer E, Roulet R (eds) Handbuch der allgemeinen Pathologie, vol VII/I. Springer, Berlin Göttingen Heidelberg

Faith Re, Liang HJ, Murgo AJ, Plotnikoff NP (1984) Neuroimmunomodulation with enkephalin: enhancement of natural killer (NK) cell activity in vitro. Clin Immunol Immunopathol 31:412–418

Falke NE, Fisher EG (1985) Cell shape of polymorphonuclear leucocytes is influenced by opioids. Immunobiology 169:532-539

Farrar WL, Hill JM, Harel-Bellan A, Vinocour M (1987) The immune logical brain. Immunol Rev 100:361–378

Felten DL, Felten SY, Carlson SL, Olochowka JA, Livnat S (1985) Noradrenergic and peptidergic innervation of lymphoid tissue. J Immunol 135: 755s–765s

Feuserstein G, Faden AL (1982) Differential cardiovascular effects of μ, δ and κ opiate agonists at discrete hypothalamic sites in the anesthetized rat. Life Sci 31:2197–2200

Fiorica E, Spector S (1988) Opioid binding site in EL-4 thymoma cell line. Life Sci 42:199–206

Fischer EG, Falke NE (1984) β-Endorphin modulates immune functions. Psychother Psychosom 42:195–204

Foreman JC, Jordan CC (1983) Histamine release and vascular changes induced by neuropeptides. Agents Actions 13:105–116

Foreman JC, Jordan CC, Piotriwski W (1982) Interaction of neurotensin with substance P receptor mediating histamine release from mast cells and the flare in human skin. Br J Pharmacol 77:531–539

Foris G, Medgyesi GA, Gyimesi E, Hanck M (1984) Met-enkephalin induced alterations of marcrophage functions. Mol-Immunol 21:747–750

Foris G, Medgyesi GA, Hanck M (1986) Bidirectional effect of Met-enkephalin on macrophage effector function. Mol Cell Biochem 69:127-137

Gausas J, Paterson PY, Day ED, Del Canto MC (1982) Intact B-cell activity in essential to complete expression of experimental allergic encephalomyelitis in Lewis rats. Cell Immunol 72:360–366

Gilman SC, Schwartz JM, Milner RJ, Bloom FE, Feldman JD (1982) β-Endorphin enhances lymphocyte proliferative responses. Proc Natl Acad Sci USA 79:4226–4230

Goetzl EJ (1977) Mast cell-mediated reactions of host defense and tissue injury: the regulatory role of eosinophil polymorphonuclear leucocytes. Inflammation 2:239–256

Goetzl EJ, Payan DG (1984) Inhibition by somatostatin of the release of mediators from human basophils and rat leukemic basophils. J Immunol 133:3255–3259

Goetzl EJ, Chernov T, Renold F, Payan DG (1985) Neuropeptide regulation of the expression of immediate hypersensitivity. J Immunol 135:802s–805s

Goldstein A (1976) Opioid peptide (endorphins) in pituitary and brain. Science 193:1081–1086

Goldstein A, Tachibara S, Lowrey LI, Hunkappilar M, Hood L (1979) Dynorphin(1-13), an extraordinarily potent opioid peptide. Proc Natl Acad Sci USA 76:6666–6670

Grandison L, Guidotti A (1977) Stimulation of food intake by muscinol and β-endorphin. Neuropharmacology 19:533–536

Guillemin R, Vargo T, Rossier J, Ling N, Rivier C, Vale W, Bloom FE (1977) β-Endorphin and adrenocorticotropin are secreted concomitantly by the pituitary gland. Science 197:1367–1369

Gungor M, Genc E, Sagduyu H, Eroglu L, Koyncuoglu H (1980) Effect of chronic administration of morphine on primary immune response in mice. Experientia 36:1309–1310

Hagermark OT, Hokfelt T, Pernow B (1978) Flare and itch induced by substance P in human skin. J Invest Dermatol 71:233–235

Hambrook JM, Morgan BA, Rance MJ, Smith CFC (1976) Mode of deactivation of enkephalin by rat and human plasma and rat brain homogenates. Nature 262:782–783

Hashim GA (1978) Myelin basic protein: structure, function and antigenic determinants. Immunol Rev 39:60–107

Hashim GA, Carvalho EF, Sharpe RD (1978) Definition and synthesis of the essential amino acid sequence for experimental allergic encephalomyelitis in Lewis rats. J Immunol 121:665–670

Hazum E, Chang KJ, Cantrecasas PC (1979) Specific nonopioid receptors for β-endorphins. Nature 205:1033–1035

Hedner T, Cassuto J (1987) Opioids and opioid receptors in peripheral tissues. Scand J Gastroenterol [Suppl] 130:27–46

Heijnen CJ, Bevers A, Kavelaars C, Balieux RE (1986) Effect of α-endorphin on the antigen-induced primary antibody response of human blood B-cells in vitro. J Immunol 136:213–216

Henson PM, Murphy RC (1989) Mediators of the inflammatory process, vol 6. Elsevier Science, Amsterdam

Hickey WE, Gonatas NK, Kimura H, Wilson DB (1983) Identification and quantification of T lymphocyte subsets found in the spinal cord of the Lewis rat during acute experimental allergic encephalomyelitis. J Immunol 131:2805–2809

Holaday JW (1983) Cardiovascular consequences of endogenous opiate antagonism. Biochem Pharmacol 32:573–585

Horvath K, Graf L, Walcz E, Bodasky H, Schuler D (1985) Naloxone antagonises effect of α-gliadin on leucocyte migration in patients with coeliac disease. Lancet II:184–185

Hughes JW, Smith T, Kosterlitz H, Fothergill L, Morgan B, Morris H (1975) Identification of two related pentapeptides from the brain with potent opiate agonist activity. Nature 255:577–579

Humphrey JR, Jaques R (1954) The histamine and serotonin content of the platelets and polymorphonuclear leucocytes of various species. J Physiol 124:305–310

Janković BD, Draskoci M, Janjić M (1965) Passive transfer of "allergic" encephalomyelitis with anti-brain serum injected into lateral ventricle of brain. Nature 207:428–429

Janković BD, Marić D (1986) Modulation of in vivo immune responses by enkephalin. Clin Neuropharmacol 9 [Suppl 4]: 476–478

Janković BD, Marić D (1987a) Enkephalin and immunity. I. In vivo suppression and potentiation of humoral immune response. Ann NY Acad Sci 496:115–125

Janković BD, Marić D (1987b) Enkephalin and anaphylactic shock: modulation and prevention of shock in the rat. Immunol Lett 15:153–160

Janković BD, Marić D (1987c) Enkephalin and autoimmunity: differential effect of methionine-enkephalin on experimental allergic encephalomyelitis in Wistar and Lewis Rats. J Neurosci Res 18:88–94

Janković BD, Marić D (1988) Enkephalins modulate in vivo immune reactions through δ- and μ-opioid receptors. Ann NY Acad Sci 540:691–693

Janković BD, Marić D (1990) Methionine-enkephalin inhibits adaptive transfer of experimental allergic encephalomyelitis in the rat. Int J Neurosci 51:197–199

Janković BD, Levic Z, Nikolic J, Stojisavljevic N (1989a) Intrathecal methionine-enkephalin in the treatment of multiple sclerosis (MS): a preliminary clinical trial. Int J Neurosci 48:155 (abstract)

Janković BD, Zozulya AA, Marić (1989b) Enkephalin and immunity: correlation of exogenous and endogenous opioids. Int J Neurosci 48:155 (abstract)

Jensen J, Snyderman R, Mergenhagen SE (1969) Chemotactic activity: a property of guinea pig C5-anaphylatoxin. In: Movat HZ (ed) Cellular and humoral mechanisms in anaphylaxis and allergy, Karger, New York

Johnson HM, Smith EM, Torres BA, Blalock JE (1982) Regulation of the in vitro antibody response by neuroendocrine hormones. Proc Natl Acad Sci USA 79:4171–4174

Kabat EA, Wolf A, Bezer AE (1947) The rapid production of acute disseminated encephalomyelitis in rhesus monkeys by injection of heterologous and homologous brain tissue with adjuvants. J Exp Med 85:117–130

Kamikawa Y, Shima Y (1983) Pharmacological characterization of the opioid receptors in the submucosus plexus of the guinea-pig oesophagus. Br J Pharmacol 78:693–699

Kay NE, Allen J, Morley JE (1984) Endorphins stimulate normal human peripheral blood lymphocyte natural killer activity. Life Sci 53:53–59

Kayashima K, Koga T, Onove K (1976) Role of T-lymphocytes in adjuvant arthritis.I.Evidence for the regulatory function of thymus-derived cells in the induction of the disease. J Immunol 117:1878–1882

Kies MW, Alvord EC (1959) Encephalolitogenic activity in guinea-pigs of water soluble protein fractions of nervous tissue. In: Keis MW, Alvord EC (eds) Allergic encephalomyelitis. Thomas, Springfied, pp 293–299

Koff WC, Dunegan MA (1985) Modulation of macrophage-mediated tumoricidal activity by neuropeptides and neurohormones. J Immunol 135:350–354

Kromer WV, Holtt V, Scmidt H, Herz A (1981) Release of immunoreactive dynorphin from the isolated guinea pig small intestine is reduced during peristaltic activity. Neurosci Lett 25:53–56

Lewis T (1927) The blood vessels of the human skin and their responses. Shaw, London

Loh HH, Tseng LF, Wei E, Li CH (1976) β-Endorphin is a potent analgesic agent. Proc Natl Acad Sci USA 73:2895–2898

Lolait SJ, Lin ATW, Toh BH, Funder JW (1984) Immunoreactive β-endorphin in a subpopulation of mouse spleen macrophages. J Clin Invest 73:277–280

Lolait SJ, Clements JA, Marwick AJ, Cheng C, McNaully M (1986) Pro-opiomelanocortin messenger ribonucleic acid and posttranslational processing of β-endorphin in spleen macrophages. J Clin Invest 77:1776–1779

Lopker A, Abood LG, Hoss W, Lionetti FJ (1980) Stereo-selective muscarinic, acetylcholine and opiate receptors in human phagocytic leucocytes. Biochem Pharmacol 29:1361–1365

Macfarlane RG (1973) Hemostatic mechanisms in tissue injury. In: Zweifach BW, Grant L, McCluskey RT (eds) The inflammatory process, vol II, Academic Press, New York, pp 335–362

Madden IV, Akil H, Patrick L, Bershus JD (1977) Stress induced parallel changes in central opioid levels and pain responsiveness in the rat. Nature 256:358–360

Mandler RN, Biddison WE, Mandler S, Serate SA (1986) β-Endorphin augments the cytolytic activity and interferon production of natural killer cells. J Immunol 136:934–939

Marić D, Janković BD (1987a) Enkephalin and immunity. II. In vivo modulation of cell mediated immunity. Ann NY Acad Sci 496:126–136

Marić D, Janković BD (1987b) Methionine-enkephalin acts via δ receptors on humoral immune response in mice. Fed Proc 46:1446

Marić D, Janković BD (1988) Therapeutic effect of methionine-enkephalin on experimental allergic encephalomyelitis (EAE). FASEB J 2:A486

Mathews PM, Froelich CJ, Sibbitt WL, Bankhurst AD (1983) Enhancement of natural cytotoxicity by β-endorphin. J Immunol 130:1658–1662

McCain HW, Lanster IB, Bilotta J (1986) Modulation of human T-cell suppressor activity by β-endorphin and glycil-L-glutamine. Int J Immunopharmacol 8:443–446

McDonough RJ, Madden JJ, Falek A, Shaker DA, Pline M, Gordon D, Bokos P, Kochale JC, Mendelson J (1980) Alteration of T- and null-cell frequencies in the peripheral blood of human opiate addicts: in vivo evidence for opiate receptor sites on T-lymphocytes. J Immunol 125:2539–2543

Mehrishi JN, Mills IJ (1983) Opiate receptors on lymphocytes and platelets in man. Clin Immunol Immunopathol 27:240–249

Meites J (1980) Interactions between hypothalamic factors and pituitary function. Fed Proc 39:2888-2940

Menkin V (1940) Dynamics of inflammation. Macmillan, New York

Metchnikoff E (1893) Lectures on the comparative pathology of inflammation. Kegan Paul, London

Meyerson BJ, Terenius L (1977) β-Endorphin and male sexual behavior. Eur J Pharmacol 42: 191–192

Monstein HJ, Folksson R, Terenius L (1986) Proenkephalin-like mRNA in human leukemia leukocytes and CNS-tissues. Life Sci 39:2237–2241

Morice A, Unwin R, Sever PS (1983) Vasoactive intestinal peptide causes bronchodilatation and protects against histamine induced bronchoconstriction in asthmatic subjects. Lancet II:1225–1227

Mosnaim AD, Wolf ME, Chevesich J, Callaghan OH, Diamond S (1985) Plasma methionine-enkephalinephalin levels: a biological marker for migraine? Headache 25:259–261

Movat HZ (ed) (1971) Inflammation, immunity and hypersensitivity. Harper and Row, New York

Nachman RL, Polley M (1979) The platelet as an inflammatory cell. In: Weissmann G, Samuelson B, Paoletti R (eds) Advances in inflammation research, vol I. Raven, New York, pp 169–173

Numa S (1984) Opioid peptide precursors and their genes. In: Udenfriend S, Meierhofer J (eds) Opioid peptides: biology, chemistry and genetics, Academic Press, New York, pp 1–23

Orgad S, Cohen I (1974) Autoimmune encephalomyelitis: activation of thymus lymphocytes against syngeneic brain antigens in vitro. Science 183:1083–1085

Oyama T, Ishihara H, Kudo T, Matsuki A (1983) Effects of hemorrhagic shock and endotoxin shock on plasma levels of β-endorphon and β-lipotropin. In: Lefer AH, Schumer W (eds) Molecular and cellular aspects of shock and trauma, Liss, New York, p 185

Paterson PY (1960) Transfer of allergic encephalomyelitis in rats by means of lymph node cells. J Exp Med 111:119–136

Paterson PY, Day ED, Whitacre CC (1981) Neuroimmune diseases: effector cell response and immunoregulatory mechanisms. Immunol Rev 55:89–120

Paterson SJ, Robson LE, Kosterlitz HW (1984) Opioid receptors. In: Udenfriend, Meierhofer J (eds) The peptides: analysis, synthesis and biology, Academic Press, London, pp 147–190

Payan DG, Levine JD, Goetzl EJ (1984) Modulation of immunity and hypersensitivity by sensory neuropeptides. J Immunol 132:1601–1604

Pearson CM (1959) Development of arthritis, periarthritis and periostitis in rats given adjuvants. Proc Soc Exp Biol Med 91:95–101

Pearson CM, Wood FD (1959) Studies of polyarthritis and other lesions induced in rats by injections of mycobacterial adjuvant. I. General clinical and pathologic characteristics and some modifying factors. Arthrit Rheumat 2:440–459

Pearson J, Brandeis L, Simon E, Hiller J (1980) Radiography of binding of tritiated diprenorphine to opiate receptors in the rat. Life Sci 26:1047–1052

Pernow B (1985) Role of tachykinins in neurogenic inflammation. J Immunol 135:812s–815s

Pert CB, Snyder SH (1973) Opiate receptor: demonstration in nervous tissue. Science 179:1011–1014

Plotnikoff NP, Wybran J, Nimeh NF, Miller GC (1986) Methionine-enkephalin: enhancement of T-cells in patients with Karposi sarcoma (AIDS). Psychopharmacol Bull 22:695–697

Portier P, Richet C (1902) De l'action anaphylactique de certains veins. CR Soc Biol 54:170

Possenti R, De Marco V, Cherubini, Roda LG (1983) Enkephalin-binding systems in human plasma. Neurochem Res 8:423–432

Prete P, Levin ER, Pedram A (1986) The in vitro effects of endogenous opiates on natural killer cells, antigen-specific cytolytic T cells, and T-cell subsets. Exp Neurol 92:349–359

Puppo F, Corsini G, Mangini P, Bottaro L, Barreca T (1985) Influence of β-endorphin on phytohemagglutinin-induced lymphocyte proliferation and on expression of mononuclear cell surface antigens in vitro. Immunopharmacology 10:119–125

Roda LG, Roscetti G, Possenti R, Venturelli F, Vita F (1986) Control mechanisms in the enzyme hydrolysis adrenal released enkephalin. In: Plotnikoff NP, Faith RE, Murgo AJ, Good RA (eds) Enkephalins and endorphins. Plenum, New York, pp 17–34

Rossier J, French ED, Rivier C, Ling N, Guillemin R, Bloom FE (1977) Foot-shock induced stress increases β-endorphin levels in blood but not brain. Nature 270:618–620

Rossle R (1923) Referat über Entzündung. Verh Dtsch Ges Pathol 27:152

Ruff M, Wahl SM, Mergenhagen S, Pert CB (1985) Opiate receptor-mediated chemotaxis of human monocytes. Neuropeptides 5:363–366

Sanyal RK, West GB (1958) Anaphylactic shock in the albino rat. J Physiol (Lond) 142:571–575

Schade H (1923) Die Physikochemie der Entzündung. Verh Dtsch Ges Pathol 19:69

Schiller PW (1984) Conformational analysis of enkephalin and conformational activity relationships. In: Undenfriend N, Meierhofer J (eds) The peptides: analysis, synthesis and biology. Academic Press, New York, pp 219–268

Schweigerer L, Schmidt W, Techemacher, Gramsch C (1985) β-Endorphin: surface binding and internalization in thymoma cells. Proc Natl Acad Sci USA 82:5751–5754

Sharp BM, Keane WE, Suh HJ, Gekker G, Tsukayama D, Peteron DK (1985) Opioid peptides rapidly stimulate superoxide production by human polymorphonuclear leukocytes and macrophages. Endocrinology 117:793–795

Simkins CO, Dickey CA, Fink MP (1984) Human neutrophil migration is enhanced by β-endorphin. Life Sci 34:2251–2255

Smith EM, Blalock JE (1981) Human lymphocyte production of corticotropin and endorphin-like substances: association with leukocyte interferon. Proc Natl Acad Sci USA 78:7530–7534

Smith EM, Johnson NM, Blalock JE (1984) Lymphocytes: peripheral source and target for endogenous opiates. In: Fraioli F, Mazzetti M (eds) Opioid peptides in the periphery. Elsevier, Amsterdam, p 129

Smith EM, Harbour-McMenamin D, Blalock JE (1985) Lymphocyte production of endorphins and endorphin-mediated immunoregulatory activity. J Immunol 135:779s–782s

Smith EM, Morrill AC, Meyer WJ, Blalock JE (1986) Corticotropin releasing factor induction of leukocyte derived immunoreactive ACTH and endorphins. Nature 321:881–882

Smith GD, Griffin JF (1978) Conformation of (Leu5) enkephalin from X-ray diffraction: features important for recognition of opiate receptor. Science 199:1214–1216

Spector WG (1979) The macrophage and its derivatives. In:Weissmann G, Samuelsson B, Paoletti R (eds) Advances in inflammation research, vol I. Raven, New York, pp 113–116

Spisani S, Traniello S (1979) Effect of mediators of inflammation on human neutrophil motility. In: Weissmann G, Samuelsson B, Paoletti R (eds) Advances in inflammation research, vol I. Raven, New York, pp 237–245

Sullivan TJ, Parker CW (1976) Pharmacologic modulation of inflammatory mediator release by rat mast cells. Am J Pathol 85:437–463

Terenius L (1973) Stereospecific interaction between narcotic analgesics and a synaptid plasma membrane fraction of rat cerebral cortex. Acta Pharmacol Toxicol (Kbh) 32:317–320

Tharp MD, Thirlby R, Sullivan TJ (1984) Gastrin induces histamine release from human cutaneous mast cells. J Allergy Immunol 74:159–165

Theoharides TC, Douglas WW (1981) Mast cell histamine secretion in response to somatostatin analogues: structural considerations. Eur J Pharmacol 73:131–136

Traugott U (1985) Characterization and distribution of lymphocyte subpopulations in multiple sclerosis plaques versus autoimmune demyelination lesions. Springer Semin Immunopathol 8:71–95

Valette A, Reme JM, Pontonnier G, Cros J (1980) Specific binding for opiate-like drugs in the placenta. Biochem Pharmacol 29:2657–2662

Van Epps DE, Saland L (1984) β-Endorphin and Met-enkephalin stimulate human peripheral blood mononuclear cell chemotaxis. J Immunol 132:3046–3053

Van Epps DE, Durant DA, Potter JW (1983) Migration of human helper-inducer T cells in response to supernatants from con A- stimulated suppressor cytotoxic T cells. J Immunol 131:697–700

Vassalli P, McCluskey RT (1971) Delayed hypersensitivity. In: Movat HZ (ed) Inflammation, immunity and hypersensitivity. Harper and Row, New York, pp 180–234

Virchow R (1858) Die Cellularpathologie in ihrer Begründung auf physiologische und pathologische Gewebelehre. Hirschwald, Berlin

Ward PA (1969) Cleavage products C3 and C5 with chemotactic activity for neutrophils.In: Movat HZ (ed) Cellular and humoral mechanisms in anaphylaxis and allergy. Karger, New York

Weissmann G, Korchak NM, Daniel Perez H, Smolen JE, Goldstein IN, Hoffstein ST (1979) Leukocytes as secretory organs of inflammation. In: Weissmann G, Samuelsson B, Paoletti R (eds) Advances in inflammation research, vol I. Raven, New York, pp 112

Wells JV (1982) Immune mechanisms in tissue damage. In: Stites DP, Stobo JD, Fudenberg HH, Wells JV (eds) Basic and clinical immunology. Lange Medical, Los Altos, pp 132–151

Wilhelm DL (1973) Chemical mediators. In: Zweifach BW, Grant L, McCluskey RT (eds) The inflammatory process. Academic Press, New York, pp 251–301

Willoughby DA (1973) Mediation of increased vascular permeability in inflammation. In: Zweifach BW, Grant L, McCluskey RT (eds) The inflammatory process, Academic Press, New York, pp 303–331

Wybran J (1985) Enkephalins and endorphins: activation molecules for the immune system and natural killer activity. Neuropeptides 5:371–374

Wybran J, Apelboom T, Famaey JP, Goavaerts A (1979) Suggestive evidence for receptors for morphine and methionine-enkephalin on normal human blood T-lymphocytes. J Immunol 123:1068–1070

Yamasaki Y, Shimamura O, Kizu A, Nakagawa N, Ijichi H (1983) Interactions of morphine with PGE_1, isoproterenol, dopamine and aminophylline in rat mast cells, their effect on lgE-mediated ^{14}C-serotonin release. Agents Actions 13:21–28

Zurawski G, Benedik M, Kamb BJ, Abrams JS, Zurawski SM, Lee FD (1986) Activation of mouse T-helper cells induces abundant preproenkephalin mRNA synthesis. Science 232:772–775

Interactions of Neuropeptides and Cytokines

T. K. Hughes Jr. and R. Chin

Introduction

An abundance of data has accumulated which strongly suggests that a linkage exists between the immune and neuroendocrine systems in vertebrates (Fischer and Falke 1984; Blalock 1985, 1989; Blalock and Smith 1985; Weigent and Blalock 1987; Dunn 1989; Smith 1991; Weigent and Blalock, Janković and Marić, both in this volume) and in invertebrates (Stefano 1989; Stefano et al. 1991). Many of the reports demonstrate that the two systems, in communicating with each other, produce and respond to similar signal molecules, i.e., cytokines and neuropeptides. The data also suggest that there is an interplay between these substances in the autoregulatory process of the immune system. More specifically, neuropeptides have been shown to effect immune responses through their influence on cytokine production and action. Conversely, cytokines are known to induce or influence the production of peptidergic messenger substances. The importance of these interactions is underscored by our recent demonstration that immune and nervous system interactions are conserved in organisms that are evolutionarily diverse from humans. For example, we have shown that opioids and monokines induce similar activities in immunocytes from a mollusc that is 500 million years divergent from humans (Fig. 1; Hughes et al. 1990; Stefano et al. 1991).

This chapter describes recent findings that demonstrate the interactions and cascades between cytokines and neuropeptides and the consequences of these interactions. We address primarily some representative reports that have become available over the past 4–5 years since earlier reviews on the subject are available (Fischer and Falke 1984; Blalock 1985, 1989; Blalock and Smith 1985; Lumpkin 1987; Stefano 1989; Dunn 1989; Smith 1991; Hughes 1992). Specifically, the following "neuropeptides" are discussed with regard to their interactions with cytokines: corticotropin (ACTH), the endorphins, arginine vasopressin (AVP) and oxytocin, thyroid stimulating hormone (TSH), vasoactive intestinal peptide (VIP), and substance P (SP). The cytokines in question include interleukins-1 and -2 (IL-1, IL-2), interferon-γ (IFN-γ), and tumor necrosis factor-alpha (TNF-α).

Department of Microbiology, J-19, University of Texas Medical Branch, Galveston, TX 77550, USA

Scharrer et al. (Eds.)
Neuropeptides and Immunoregulation

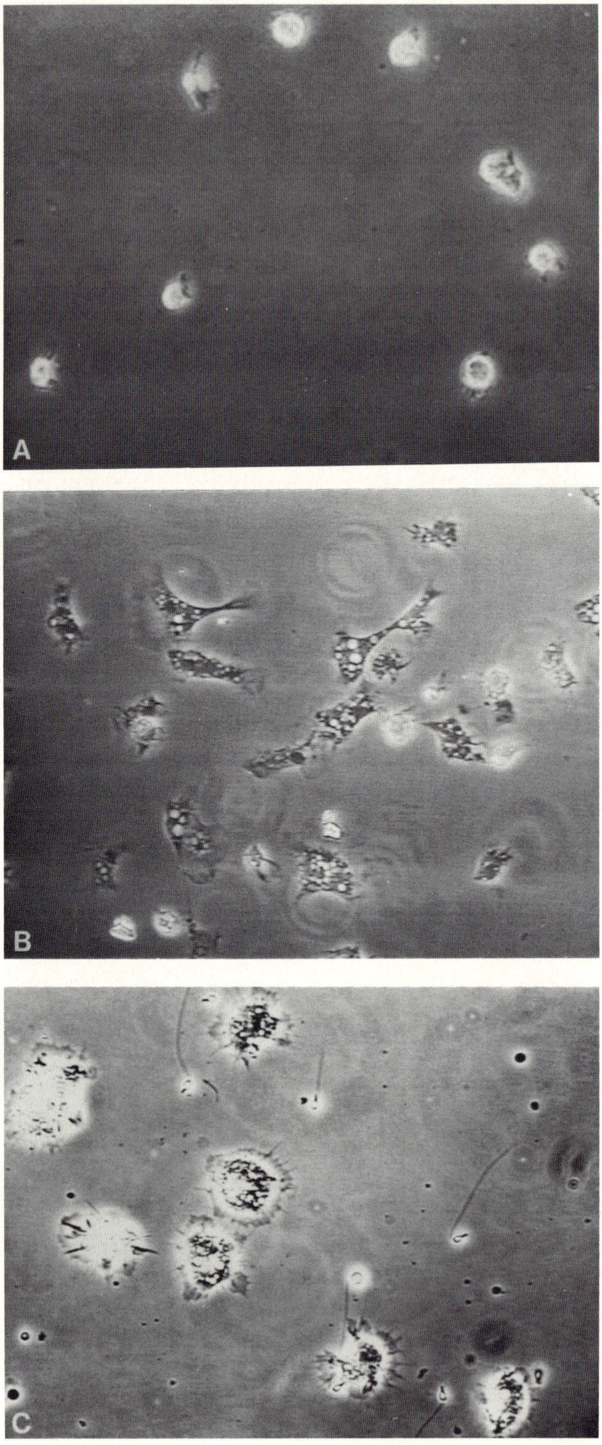

Fig. 1A–C. Conformational effects of an opioid and a cytokine on immunocytes of *Mytilus, edulis*, photomicroscopic analysis. **A** Nontreated control cells (round and small, 10 μm in diameter). **B** D-Ala^2-D-Met^5-enkephalin treated cells (10^{-11} *M*, polymorphic response). **C** Tumor necrosis factor treated cells (1 U/ml, rounded and polymorphic cells)

Corticotropin

ACTH has probably been the most intensely studied hormone in the immune and neuroendocrine systems. Produced and processed from pro-opiomelanocortin (POMC) in the pituitary gland (Norman and Litwack 1987), the hypothalamus (Krieger 1983), and lymphocytes (Blalock 1989), it has been shown to play a major role in biological and environmentally induced stress responses (Norman and Litwack 1987). It also affects immune-related phenomena such as production of antibody (Johnson et al. 1982a).

ACTH and Interleukins-1 and -2

IL-1 was one of the earliest described cytokines. Primarily produced by monocytes, it participates in responses such as induction of fever, cartilage breakdown, bone resorption, activation of T- and B-lymphocytes, and induction of fibroblast and bone marrow stem cell proliferation (reviewed by Dower et al. 1992). IL-2 was originally found in the supernatant fluids of mitogen-stimulated lymphocytes. It is produced primarily by helper T-cells and participates in responses such as T-cell growth, cytokine secretion, lymphocyte cytotoxic activity, antibody production, macrophage cytocidal activity, and lymphokine-activated killer cell activity (reviewed by Pontzer et al. 1992).

Perhaps the most thorougly studied association between a neuropeptide and a cytokine is that for ACTH and the interleukins (for reviews see Lumpkin 1987; Blalock 1989). Alvarez-Mon et al. (1985) reported that optimal growth and Ig synthesis occur in human B-lymphocytes in vitro when ACTH is combined with IL-2. ACTH has no activity when used alone. A direct induction of ACTH by IL-1 on cultured AtT-20 pituitary tumor cells occurs (Woloski et al. 1985). IL-1 was found to be equipotent to the classical ACTH inducer combination of corticotropin-releasing factor (CRF) and arginine-vasopressin. The results suggest that a combination of immunocytes, the pituitary, and hypothalamic neurons may play a role in regulating host defenses.

The POMC product α-melanocyte stimulating hormone (α- MSH) has been shown to inhibit IL-1 induced synthesis of acute-phase proteins and neutrophilia in vivo (Robertson et al. 1986). That α-MSH is incapable of modifying the co-mitogenic influence of IL-1 on thymocytes or an IL-1 responsive cell line suggests that IL-1 and α-MSH do not compete for the same receptors. In 1986 Besedovsky et al. reported that IL-1 administered in subpyrogenic doses to mice and rats results in an increase in blood levels of ACTH. Tumor necrosis factor (TNF) IL-2, and IFN-γ have no effects on ACTH levels. The effect is probably due directly to IL-1 and not to a secondary T-cell product since athymic nude mice also produce ACTH following a similar treatment.

IL-1 induced ACTH release from anterior pituitary cell cultures occurs through its induction of CRF (Berkenbosch et al. 1987) since IL-1 induced ACTH levels are reduced in the presence of anti-CRF. Blockage of hypothalamic neurons by colchicine results in a decrease in CRF in the median eminence, suggesting an enhanced release. Similar to this report, Uehara et al. (1987a) showed in rats that IL-1 induced ACTH secretion in vivo occurs through its induction of CRF since anti-CRF administered in conjunction with IL-1 prevents it. Uehara et al. (1987b) also reported on the differential abilities of IL-1α and IL-1β to increase ACTH levels in vivo. In rats they found that IL-1β but not IL-1α induces ACTH, suggesting a different spectrum of biological actions for the two molecules. IL-1 did not have any direct effect on ACTH secretion in primary rat anterior pituitary cells (Uehara et al. 1987c). In addition, these authors demonstrated a synergistic interaction with CRF.

In 1988, Boyle et al. reported that IL-1 prevents the loss of pituitary cell responsiveness to the β-adrenergic agonist 1-isoproteronol. They showed that in the presence of IL-1 normal rat anterior pituitary cells maintain an ACTH response to the β-adrenergic agonist which otherwise would have been shifted to an α-adrenergic response. It has been suggested that the anti-inflammatory action of IL-1α and-β and TNF-α in rats might be mediated through the pituitary adrenal axis (Nakamura et al. 1988). Using a model in which hind paw edema was induced by carageenan in rats, it was found that both IL-1 and TNF inhibit the edema, in part through pituitary-adrenal axis stimulation since adrenalectomized rats exhibited reduced anti-edema activity. The administration of ACTH and cytokine-containing supernatants also results in a synergistic interaction in the release of corticosterone in rats treated with endotoxin or under psychoneurogenic stress (Torres-Aleman et al. 1988).

An evaluation of the influence of IL-2 associated immunotherapy in patients for changes in ACTH and corticotropin-releasing hormone (CRH) levels (Denicoff et al. 1989) showed that the levels of these hormones are increased 4 h after the administration of IL-2 or IL-2 plus lymphokine-activated killer cells. It was further shown that a second course of IL-2 given to these patients results in an even further increase in these neuropeptide levels. Smith et al. (1989) showed the presence of an IL-2 receptor α-chainlike molecule on the surface of pituitary cells. The functionality of this receptor was implied by the finding that pituitary cells released ACTH following stimulation with IL-2. Furthermore, synthesis of aldosterone in adrenal glomerulosa cells stimulated with ACTH is potentiated by IL-1 (Natarajan et al. 1989). The release of hormones from normal rat anterior pituitary cells after treatment with cytokines has also been reported (Kehrer et al. 1989). Dispersed rat anterior pituitary cells were stimulated for 24 h with IL-1α. ACTH levels measured 3 days later were found to be increased in dose-dependent fashion. In contrast, TNF-α failed to stimulate ACTH secretion. Rat pituitaries also produce ACTH following treatment with thymosin (McGillis et al. 1988). Similarly plasma levels of ACTH and catecholamines in rats increase after IL-1α or β administration. IL-1β is generally more effective than IL-1α in causing the ACTH increase especially after administration by intracerebroventricular injection (Rivier et al. 1989a).

There is also evidence for catecholamines playing a role in IL-1 induction of ACTH in rats (Weidenfield et al. 1989). The neurotoxin 6-hydroxydopamine and α_1-adrenergic antagonist were shown to inhibit IL-1 induction of ACTH, suggesting that central adrenergic transmission is involved in the adrenocortical response to IL-1. Opp et al. (1989) investigated the effects of CRF on IL-1 induced pyrogen effects and non-REM sleep in rabbits. They found that IL-1 enhanced eye movements are inhibited by CRF, and that fever is reduced after several hours. Infectious agents such as Newcastle disease virus stimulate the pituitary adrenal axis possibly through the induction of IL-1 production by peripheral lymphocytes (Besedovsky and Rey 1989). Activation of the hypothalamic-pituitary-adrenal axis by a bacterial product, endotoxin, occurs through a mechanism involving IL-1 receptors, and the effect of IL-1β but not-α on ACTH secretion in the mouse can be partially blocked by MSH (Rivier et al. 1989b).

IL-1 and -6 but not IL-2 can stimulate the release of ACTH from AtT-20 pituitary cells after a latent period (Fukata et al. 1989). Further, while nontreated cells were relatively insensitive to CRF, they showed a significant response following treatment with IL-1β. In addition to IL-1, pituitary cells from patients with Cushing's syndrome respond to thymosin fraction 5, IFN-γ and granulocyte colony-stimulating factor by producing ACTH (Malarkey and Zvara 1989). The relative efficacy of IL-1 or TNF on ACTH production in rats has been compared (Sharp et al. 1989), and TNF appears to be a potent secretagogue for ACTH in the plasma. It appeared that IL-1 and TNF have complementary modes of action. However, the target of TNF action appeared to be peripheral to the CNS and pituitary in contrast to that of IL-1. Mason and Van Epps (1989) reported on the effects of MSH and ACTH on IL-1α and TNF-α induced chemotaxis. They found that both peptides effectively inhibit migration of neutrophils into subcutaneously implanted sponges in the mouse, suggesting that these neuropeptides may be important inflammatory regulators.

In 1990 Gwosdow et al. reported that pituitary ACTH levels rise in rats following IL-1 administration. A parallel rise was noted in plasma levels and was abrogated by hypophysectomy. IL-1 also mediates CRF-induced secretion of β-endorphin by lymphocytes in vivo (Kavelaars et al. 1990a). Acute administration of IL-1α and β stimulates hypothalamic CRF gene expression and release, which subsequently stimulates POMC gene expression and ACTH release in the anterior pituitary (Suda et al. 1990).

IL-2 at picomolar concentrations induces the release of ACTH from intact portions of rat anterior pituitary glands 1 h after perfusion. The release of several other hormones is affected, indicating that IL-2 may be an important messenger from lymphocytes which exerts a direct paracrine effect on the pituitary (Karanth and McCann 1991). IL-1 and IL-2 in cultured rat adrenal cells increase corticosterone levels (Tominaga et al. 1991). Corticosterone production is accompanied by both intracellular and extracellular cAMP and prostaglandin accumulation which is potentiated by ACTH. Weiss et al. (1991) reported that α-MSH , introduced simultaneously into the cerebroventricular system with IL-1, totally blocks elevation of plasma ACTH and corticosterone levels. In addition, they showed that it suppresses IL-1 enhanced natural killer (NK) activity. Since IL-1 promotes production of α-MSH, the results suggest that there is a negative feedback. IL-1β, while acting in conjunction with other products of the immune system to modulate adrenal cortisol production, does not directly influence human fetal steroidogenesis but acts through ACTH induction (Harlin and Parker 1991). Finally, Navarra et al. (1991) reported that IL-1 and IL-6 induced release of CRH-41 from rat hypothalami occurs through the eicosanoid cyclo-oxygenase pathway.

ACTH and IFN-γ

IFN-γ is produced primarily by T-lymphocytes in response to antigenic or mitogenic stimuli. IFN-γ has several roles including induction of antiviral activity, activation of macrophages, induction of class II antigen, and inhibition of cell proliferation (reviewed by Vankelecom and Billiau 1992).

The initial demonstration of the effects of ACTH on IFN-γ production was that of Johnson et al. (1984). They found that ACTH inhibited the production of IFN-γ induced by the lectin phytohemagglutinin. Similarly, Koff and Dunegan (1985, 1986) found that ACTH inhibits IFN-γ activation of macrophages to a cytocidal state. This includes macrophage-mediated cytolysis of transformed and virus-infected target cells. ACTH significantly inhibits the chemoluminescence associated with blood monocytes treated with concanavalin A (an IFN-γ inducer; Hanmann et al. 1988). It also decreases the ability of IFN-γ treated macrophages to bind ^{125}I-labeled TNF, suggesting a decrease in IFN-γ induced TNF receptors (Bermudez et al. 1990). From these studies, it generally appears that ACTH has an inhibitory effect on responses related to IFN-γ. In contrast it was recently demonstrated that ACTH itself induces and, in addition, potentiates IFN-γ induced production of TNF from monocytes (Hughes and Smith 1989). Vankelecom et al. in 1990 showed that pretreatment of normal rat anterior pituitary cells with IFN-γ prevents the stimulation of ACTH secretion by CRF. TNF-α and IL-6 were also shown to inhibit this release but with a less pronounced effect.

ACTH and TNF

TNF is a cytokine produced primarily by macrophages, monocytes, NK cells, and astrocytes in response to infectious and inflammatory stimuli. TNF has numerous activities, including mediation of cachexia, cytotoxic effects against tumor cells, induction of antiviral activity, and activation of macrophages (reviewed by Martin and Tracey 1992).

In 1987 Besedovsky and del Rey tested TNF for its ability to induce ACTH and corticosterone output. In contrast to IL-1, TNF lacked the ability to induce such effects. However, TNF was found to induce the release of ACTH (in addition to other hormones) from fragments of rat anterior pituitaries or dispersed anterior pituitary cells in vitro (Milenkovic et al. 1989). They found that the doses of TNF used are roughly equivalent to those found in the plasma during infection suggestive of pathophysiological significance. Rettori et al. (1989) investigated the hypothalamic action of TNF in vivo. Only at the highest level of the cytokine used was a small but significant rise in plasma ACTH levels observed. In contrast, it was shown that TNF administered to rats significantly enhances the plasma levels of ACTH and corticosterone among other peptides (Darling et al. 1989).

In vitro ACTH could both directly induce TNF and potentiate the IFN-γ induction of TNF from the adherent fraction of peripheral blood leukocytes (Hughes and Smith 1989). In light of the results of Koff and Dunegan (1986) which showed that ACTH blocks the IFN-γ activation of monocyte cytotoxicity, this finding was unexpected since TNF is thought to be a mediator of macrophage cytotoxicity (Philip and Epstein 1986). Jaattela et al. (1990) studied the effects of TNF on the regulation of ACTH induced steroidogenesis. Measureable TNF-α was found in fetal but not adult adrenals. TNF was shown effectively to suppress the production of cortisol, suggesting that it may play a role in regulating fetal steroidogenesis. CRF could be a major mediator of the hypothalamic-pituitary-adrenal axis response to TNF (Bernardini et al. 1990). They found that TNF given intravenously in the rat stimulates plasma ACTH and corticosterone secretion in a dose-dependent fashion. This stimulation was blocked if the rats received antibody to CRF prior to TNF administration. TNF suppression of ACTH-induced cortisol synthesis has also been shown to be accompanied by a shift of the steroid secretory pattern toward androgen production (Jaattela et al. 1991).

Endorphins

The endorphins were primarily thought to be products of the CNS until it was shown that lymphocytes both produce endorphins and possess specific receptors for them (for review see Blalock 1989). Endorphins are endogenous opioids that are central to the control and perception of pain. In addition to this and several other roles, they interact with cytokines in immunoregulatory processes (for reviews see Fischer and Falke 1984; Morely et al. 1985; Blalock 1989; Dunn 1989).

Smith and Blalock (1981) found that infection of lymphocytes with Newcastle disease virus results in the release of an endorphin-like activity in addition to that of IFN-α. This finding partially explains the opiate-like side effects seen with exogenous IFN administration in mice. Koff and Dunegan (1985) also found that β-endorphin does not block the tumoricidal activity of IFN-γ treated macrophages, in contrast to ACTH and noradrenaline. They also showed that, in contrast to epinephrine and norepinephrine, β-endorphin does not suppress IFN-γ induced, macrophage-mediated lysis of herpes simplex virus infected target cells (Koff and Dunegan 1986). β-endorphin enhances the production of IFN-γ in concanavalin A stimulated human mononuclear cells (Brown and Van Epps 1986). This enhancement was not reversible by naloxone. Conversely, β-endorphin and Met-enkephalin inhibit NK and cytolytic T-cell activity (Prete et al. 1986). The effects of α-endorphin on antigen-induced primary antibody responses to ovalbumin have been studied by Heijnen et al. (1986). Responses were blocked at both the T-cell and B-cell levels. α-Endorphin lacking the N-terminal tyrosine had no effect. Thymosin fraction 5 stimulates the secretion of irβ-endorphin in mouse corticotropic tumor cells. It was also found that this fraction enhances CRF-induced β-endorphin secretion (Farah et al. 1987).

In 1987 Peterson et al. reported on the effects of β-endorphin and morphine on the production of IFN-γ from peripheral blood mononuclear cells. They found that a significant suppression was caused by both compounds, suggesting a mechanism whereby opiate addiction and stress contribute to impaired cell-mediated immunity. They also found that β-endorphin and morphine suppress production of IFN-γ by peripheral blood mononuclear cells in response to concanavalin A and varicella zoster virus. Monocytes appeared to be the primary target cells for opioids, suggesting that an opioid-triggered release of some inhibitory monocyte derived metabolite might play a role in the immunodeficiency associated with stress and narcotics. In autologous and allogenic mixed lymphocyte reactions it was found that β-endorphin but not α-endorphin augments the former but not the latter (Froelich 1987). Foster and Moore (1987) demonstrated that dynorphin enhances IFN activation of murine peritoneal macrophage tumoricidal activity while Oleson and Johnson (1988) found that opioid peptides modulate NK activity in a bimodal fashion. They also found that high NK activity was suppressed while low NK activity was enhanced. Naloxone displayed both antagonistic and direct modulatory activity in their system (Oleson and Johnson 1988). Mandler et al. (1986) also found that β-endorphin augments the cytolytic activity and, in addition, IFN production of NK cells (Mandler et al. 1988). It also potentiates IL-2 induced lymphokine-activated killer cell formation, conceivably through inhibition of adenylate cyclase activity (Beckner and Farrar 1988). It also potentiates IL-2 induced lymphokine-activated killer cell formation, conceivably through inhibition of adenylate cyclase activity (Beckner and Farrar 1988). This was also shown for somatostatin.

Cancer patients receiving IL-2 associated immunotherapy have increased levels of β-endorphin 4 h following administration. An even greater increase was noted after a second course of immunotherapy (Denicoff et al. 1989). Fagarasan et al. (1989) found that IL-1 enhances β-endorphin secretion induced by CRF and VIP, possibly through protein kinase C. IL-1 derived from $CD14^+$ monocytes mediates the effect of CRF and AVP on β-endorphin production by B-cells (Kavelaars et al. 1989). Gilmore and Weiner (1988) reported that β-endorphin enhances the production of IL-2 from mitogen-stimulated murine splenocytes and from a cloned T-cell line. This enhancement was not reversible by naloxone, suggesting that it might occur through a non-opioid receptor for β-endorphin on the lymphoid cell.

β-endorphin affects IL-1 induced IL-2 production in the lymlphoid cell line EL-4 (Bessler et al. 1990). It was shown to enhance IL-2 production in response to both IL-1α and -β, and the effect was inhibited by naloxone, suggesting an action through opioid receptors. An IL-1 dependent CRF induction of β-endorphin occurs in lymphocytes (Kavelaars et al. 1990a, b). In addition, β-endorphin potentiates lipopolysaccharide induced IL-1 secretion from bone marrow macrophages (Apte et al. 1990). They found that α-endorphin had no effect. Van-den-Bergh et al. (1991) found two opposing modes of action of β-endorphin on lymphocyte function. While β-endorphin enhances concanavalin A induced proliferation of T-cells if added 30 min prior to stimulation, the continuous presence in culture abolished the enhancement. The intracellular signaling pathways involved in the regulation of β-endorphin secretion by human peripheral blood mononuclear cells has been studied (Kavelaars et al. 1991). Fast and slow responses can be detected depending on the stimulus used. These responses appear to be mediated by protein kinase C and by a combination of protein kinase C and A activation, respectively.

Arginine Vasopressin and Oxytocin

AVP is a nonapeptide hormone produced by hypothalamic neurons. AVP plays important regulatory roles which include antidiuretic effects (Sawyer 1961), vasopressor effects (Rossi and Schrier 1986), and modulation of stress responses (Gibbs 1986). Oxytocin is structurally related to AVP and primarily promotes uterine contraction and milk ejection (Tepperman 1980).

Block et al. (1981) reported on the specific binding of ^{125}I-labeled 8-L-AVP to mononuclear phagocytes. Binding was shown to be saturable ($2.8 + 0.4$ fmol/2×10^6 cells/ml), linear with cell number, and reversible. The specificity of the binding was determined by use of a series of vasopressin analogues. AVP can replace the IL-2 requirement for IFN-γ production by Lyt-2^+ C57BL/6 mouse spleen cells (Johnson et al. 1982b). Oxytocin is also capable of replacing IL-2. The six amino acids of the N-terminal provide the helper signal based on the relative ability of AVP, oxytocin, vasotocin, and pressinoic acid to help in IFN-γ production (Johnson and Torres 1985). It was suggested that the AVP signal operates through an AVP vasopressor-type receptor on the lymphocyte. Oxytocin receptors in the rat thymic gland have also been described (Elands et al. 1988). The receptor appears to have a ligand specificity similar to that of uterine receptors.

Following their finding that AVP could provide a helper signal during IFN-γ production, evidence for a novel AVP receptor on mouse lymphocytes was described by Torres and Johnson in 1988. It was found that two V_1 vasopressor receptor antagonists that work identically on liver cells differ in their ability to block AVP effects in the lymphocyte system, while V_2 antidiuretic receptor antagonists have no effect. They also showed that a peptide complementary to

AVP blocks AVP modulation of immune function (Johnson and Torres 1988). Since AVP requires conformational flexibility for signal transduction, it was hypothesized that the complementary peptide is binding to AVP and converting it to an antagonist of its own action.

Kavelaars et al. (1989) reported that the presence of monocytes is required for AVP and CRF to induce β-endorphin. It appeared that AVP and CRF induce the monocyte to secrete IL-1, which in turn causes the B-cell to secrete β-endorphin. Studies have been performed to determine whether interleukins are involved in AVP or oxytocin release (Naito et al. 1991). These results and others (Locher et al. 1983) suggest that IL-1 increases plasma AVP and oxytocin levels in rats, and that different kinds of prostaglandins are involved in this release.

Thyrotropin

TSH, a glycoprotein hormone released from the pituitary gland, is not a neuropeptide but is controlled by one, the thyrotropin-releasing hormone (TRH). In addition to its well-established functions in the maintenance of homeostasis (Field 1986), TSH has been shown to affect the immune system and to interact with cytokines. TSH enhances MHC class II antigen expression in cultured thyrocytes. This occurs following treatment of the cells with IFN-γ (Todd et al. 1987a, b). In vitro, the cytotoxic effect of TNF for thyroid epithelial cells pretreated with IFN-γ is markedly enhanced by the presence of TSH (Taverne et al. 1987). Several reports have shown that IL-1 can induce the production of TSH. Bernton et al. (1987) demonstrated that monolayers of rat pituitary cells produce TSH following treatment with IL-1. Ex vivo experiments indicate that rat pituitaries perfused with IL-1 rapidly produce TSH in addition to other hormones (Beach et al. 1989). This rapid response suggests that IL-1 acts acutely to release preformed hormone stores. Other reports have shown that IL-1 injected into rats results in a decrease in TSH levels (Rettori et al. 1987; Dubuis et al. 1988). However, TNF induces the production of TSH from both rat hemipituitaries and dispersed anterior pituitary cells at physiological concentrations (Milenkovic et al. 1989).

Combinations of TNF with somatostatin result in enhanced TSH production. Krueger et al. (1989) demonstrated that TRH enhances the in vitro antibody response to a T-cell dependent mitogen. Presumably, this occurs through induction of TSH (see Blalock 1989). Thyrocyte HLA class II expression stimulated by TSH in the presence of IFN-γ can be suppressed by epidermal growth factor (Todd et al. 1990). A report by Harbour et al. (1990) indicates that some of the TSH regulatory activities in B-cells occur through specific bioactive receptors. TSH was further shown to affect the B-cell proliferative response to lipopolysaccharide. The effects of IFN-γ on the morphology of thyroid follicles and their expression of class II molecules has been described (Asakawa et al. 1991). IFN-γ was shown to inhibit TSH-induced morphological changes while inducing the expression of class II molecules on these cells.

Vasoactive Intestinal Peptide

VIP was first identified on the basis of its vasodilator action. It occurs widely in the intestinal and nervous systems of mammals and lower vertebrates. VIP has many activities which include suppression of gastric acid secretion, stimulation of intestinal H_2O and ion secretion, promotion of splanchnic blood flow, and induction of cyclic AMP (Norman and Litwack 1987).

With respect to its interactions with cytokines, VIP potentiates the suppressive effects of norepinephrine on the IFN-γ activation of macrophages to a tumoricidal state (Koff and Dunegan 1985). It also decreases IL-2 production in mouse lymphocytes responding to concanavalin A (Ottaway 1987). A similar inhibitory effect of VIP was shown by the decreased ability of IFN-γ to induce class II antigen expression in astrocytes obtained from rats (Frohman et al. 1988). On the other hand, Fagarasan et al. (1989) found that pretreatment of AtT-20 pituitary tumor cells with IL-1 enhances VIP-induced secretion of ACTH and β-endorphin. IFN-γ affects chloride secretion in enterocytes responding to VIP (Holmgren et al. 1989). They found that IFN-γ markedly increases the chloride secretory response of these cells to VIP. Schettini et al. (1990) found that IL-1 inhibits prolactin secretion from VIP- stimulated anterior pituitary tumor cells. In addition to its hormonal action, VIP is capable of inducing an antiviral state in HT-29 colonic tumor cells through its induction of IFN (Chelbi-Alix et al. 1990). In addition to lipopolysacchride and IL-1, VIP stimulates IL-6 release from anterior pituitary cells (Spangelo et al. 1991). In the presence of VIP and prostaglandin E_2, IL-1-α and -β increase IL-6 release without any apparent change in intra- or extracellular cAMP.

Substance P

SP is an undecapeptide belonging to a group of proteins called tachykinins. It is present in the brain, spinal ganglia, and intestine. It has been shown to have several activities, including vasodilation, pain production, salivation stimulation, and capillary permeability increases (Zadina et al. 1986; Aronin et al. 1986).

Koff and Dunegan (1985) tested the effect of SP on IFN-γ activated macrophage cytotoxic activity and found that it has no effect. On the other hand, SP was shown directly to induce the production of lymphokines in mice (Paegelow and Werner 1986) and increase IFN-γ levels in peripheral blood leukocytes treated with pokeweed mitogen (PWM) but not phytohemagglutinin (Wagner et al. 1987). SP increases tumoricidal activity of macrophages by IFN-γ independent and dependent mechanisms (Peck 1987). It also increases the proportion of macrophages able to secrete superoxide ions, suggesting a possible influence on macrophage capacity to deal with microbial infection. SP induces IL-1 in human monocytes (Lotz et al. 1988) and in murine P388D1 cells and potentiates IL-1 induced cell proliferation in BALB/3T3 cells (Kimball and Fischer 1988; Kimball et al. 1988). In PWM-treated human duodenal cell cultures, SP reduces the levels of IL-1 β but enhances the levels of IL-2 and IL-2 receptors (Hart et al. 1988). SP levels in the ascitic fluid of humans with various types of malignancy increase 10 to 140-fold following infusion with IL-2 and lymphokine-activated killer cells (Schiogolev et al. 1989). In blood monocytes, Laurentzi et al. (1990) reported that SP induces the production of IL-1 from human monocytes, but that the levels varied from culture to culture. Hart et al. (1990) reported that human duodenal mucosa, when treated with PWM and SP, responded by producing more immunoglobulin and IFN-γ after 3–4 days in culture than those treated with PWM alone. Cytokines also affect the release of SP in sympathetic neurons (Freiden and Kessler 1991). Exposure of cultures of neuronal and nonneuronal cells of sympathetic ganglia to IL-1β results in an increase in SP, but there was no effect on the peptide content of pure neuronal cultures. The increase was blocked by dexamethasone. IL-2 and TNF had no effect on SP expression.

Conclusions

The observations of neuropeptides interacting with cytokines indicate that a complex series of events occurs during basal homeostasis. The finding that these cascades and interactions are conserved in humans and reach back to invertebrates 500 million years divergent in evolution indicates the fundamental importance of these mechanisms (Fig 2). Once the systems are activated by

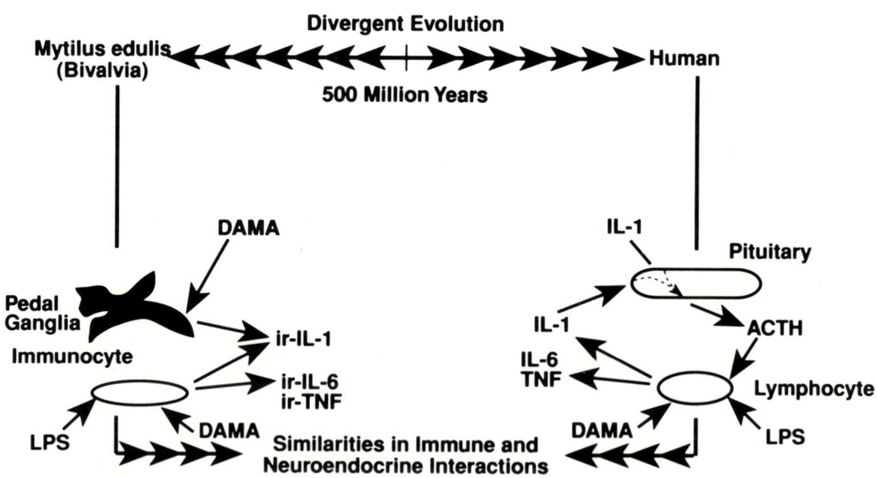

Fig. 2. Interactions between immune and nervous systems in *Mytilus edulis*, comparable to those in mammals

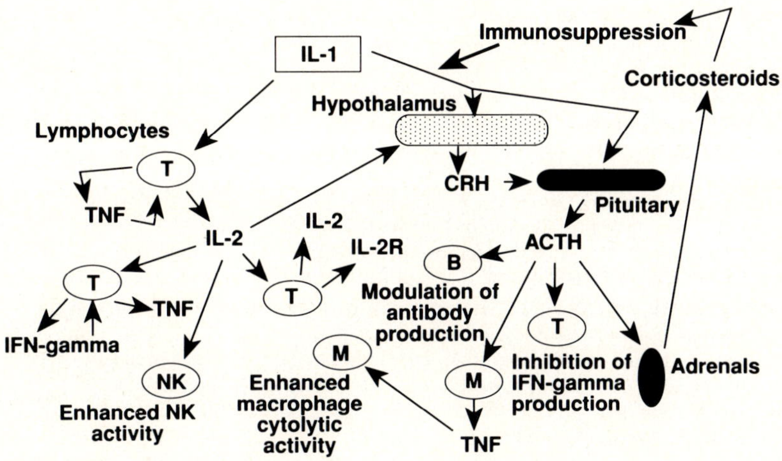

Fig. 3. Possible cascade initiated by single mediator, IL-1, in the human immune and neuroendocrine system. *T*, T-cells; *B*, B-cells; *M*, macrophages; *IL-2R*, IL-2 receptor

environmental or biological stressors, the series of events that can be envisioned to take place become even more dramatic. Studying single factors in the network of interconnecting pathways between the immune and neuroendocrine systems becomes, at best, elucidation of only a minor component. What is actually occurring, and how the shared mediators are affecting each other is a function of multiple factors and how they interact. Add to this the rhythmicity that occurs in neuroendocrine system responses and the difficulty becomes exponential (Fig 3). The potential for study in this field is therefore apparently still very broad and will undoubtedly produce additional suprising results.

References

Apte RN, Durum SK, Oppenheim JJ (1990) Opioids modulate interleukin-1 production and secretion by bone marrow macrophages. Immunol Lett 24(2):141–148

Alvarez-Mon M, Kehrl JH, Fauci AS (1985) A potential role for adrenocorticotropin in regulating human B-lymphocyte functions. J Immunol 135(6):3823–3826

Aronin N, Coslovsky R, Leeman SE (1986) Substance P and neurotensin: their roles in the regulation of anterior pituitary function. Annu Rev Physiol 48:537–549

Asakawa H, Hanafusa T, Katsura H, Miyagawa J, Otsuka A, Nakagawa C, Itoh N, Kono N, Tarui S (1991) Interferon-γ inhibits thyroid stimulating-hormone induced morphological changes and induces the expression major histocompatability complex class II antigens in thyroid follicles in suspension culture. Endocrinology 128(3):1409–1413

Beach JE, Smallridge RC, Kinzer CA, Bernton EW, Holaday JW (1989) Rapid release of multiple hormone from rat pituitaries perfused with recombinant interleukin-1. Life Sci 44(1):1–7

Beckner SK, Farrar WL (1988) Potentiation of lymphokine-activated killer cell differentiation and lymphocyte proliferation by stimulation of protein kinase C or inhibition of adenylate cyclase. J Immunol 140(1):208–214

Berkenbosch F, van Oers J, del Rey A, Tilders F, Besedovsky H (1987) Corticotropin-releasing factor-producing neurons in the rat activated by interleukin-1. Science 238(4826):524–526

Bermudez LE, Wu M, Young LS (1990) Effect of stress-related hormones on macrophage receptors and response to tumor necrosis factor. Lymphokine Res 9(2):137–145

Bernadini R, Kamilaris TC, Calogero AE, Johnson EO, Gomez MT, Gold PW, Chrousos GP (1990) Interactions between tumor necrosis factor-α, hypothalamic corticotropin releasing hormone, and adrenocorticotropin secretion in the rat. Endocrinology 126(6):2876–2881

Bernton EW, Beach JE, Holaday JW, Smallridge RC, Fein HG (1987) Release of multiple hormones by a direct action of interleukin-1 on pituitary cells. Science 238(4826):519–521

Besedovsky H, del Rey A (1987) Neuroendocrine and metabolic responses induced by interleukin-1. J Neurosci Res 18(1):172–178

Besedovsky H, del Rey A (1989) Mechanism of virus induced stimulation of the hypothalamus-pituitary-adrenal axis. J Steroid Biochem 34(1–6):235–239

Besedovsky H, del Ray A, Sorkin E, Dinarello CA (1986) Immunoregulatory feedback between interleukin-1 and glucocorticoid hormones. Science 233(4764):652–654

Bessler H, Sztein MB, Serrate SA (1990) α-Endorphin modulation of IL-2 induced IL-2 production. Immunopharmacology 19:5–14

Blalock JE (1985) Proopiomelanocortin derived peptides in the immune system. Clin Endocrinol 22(6):823–827

Blalock JE (1989) A molecular basis for bidirectional communication between the immune and neuroendocrine systems. Physiol Rev 69(1):1–32

Blalock JE, Smith EM (1985) A complete regulatory loop between the immune and neuroendocrine systems. Fed Proc 44:101–111

Block L, Locher R, Tenschert W, Siegenthaler W, Hofmann T, Mettler R, Vetter W (1981) 125-I-8-L-Arginine vasopressin binding to human mononuclear phagocytes. J Clin Invest 68: 374–381

Boyle M, Yamamoto G, Chen M, Rivier J, Vale W (1988) Interleukin-1 prevents loss of corticotropic responsiveness to β-adrenergic stimulation in vitro. Proc Natl Acad Sci USA 85(15): 5556–5560

Brown SL, Van Epps DE (1986) Opioid peptides modulate production of interferon-γ by human mononuclear cells. Cell Immunol 103(1):19–26

Chelbi-Alix MK, Boissard C, Rosselin G, Thang MN (1990) Vasoactive intestinal peptide induces 2′,5′ oligoadenylate synthetase and antiviral state in cells of HT-29 colonic cancer, C R Acad Sci III 310(5):147–153

Darling G, Goldstein DS, Stull R, Gorschboth CM, Norton JA (1989) Tumor necrosis factor: immune endocrine interaction. Surgery 106(6):1155–1160

Denicoff D, Durkin TM, Lotze MT, Quinlan PE, Davis CL, Listwak SJ, Rosenberg SA, Rubinow DR (1989) The neuroendocrine effects of interleukin-2 treatment. J Clin Endocrinol Metab 89(2): 402–410

Dower SK, Bird TA, Sims JE (1992) Interleukin-1. Adv Neuroimmunol 2:1–16

Dubuis JM, Dayer JM, Siegrest-Kaiser CA, Burger AG (1988) Human recombinant interleukin-1-β decreases plasma thyroid hormone and thyroid stimulating hormone levels in rats. Endocrinology 123(5):2175–2181

Dunn AJ (1989) Psychoneuroimmunology for the psychoneuroendocrinologist: a review of nervous system–immune system interactions. Psychoneuroendocrinology 14(4):251–274

Elands J, Annelies R, DeKloet ER (1988) Oxytocin receptors in the rat thymic gland. Eur J Pharmacol 151(2):345–346

Fagarsaan MO, Eskay R, Axelrod J (1989) Interleukin-1 potentiates the secretion of β-endorphin induced by secretagogues in a mouse pituitary cell line (AtT-20). Proc Natl Acad Sci USA 86(6): 2070–2073

Farah JM Jr, Hall NR, Bishop JF, Goldstein AL, O'Donohue TL (1987) Thymosin fraction 5 stimulates secretion of immunoreactive β-endorphin in mouse corticotropic tumor cells. J Neurosci Res 18(1):140–146

Field JB (1986) Mechanism of action of thyrotropin. In: Ingbar SH, Braverman LE (eds) The thyroid, a fundamental and clinical text. Lippincott, Philadelphia

Fischer EG, Falke NE (1984) β-endorphin modulates immune functions. A review. Psychother Psychosom 42(1–4):195–204

Foster JS, Moore RN (1987) Dynorphin and related opioid peptides enhance tumoricidal activity mediated by murine peritoneal macrophages. J Leukoc Biol 42(2):171–174

Freiden M, Kessler JA (1991) Cytokine regulation of substance P expression in sympathetic neurons. Proc Natl Acad Sci USA 88(8):3200–3203

Froelich CJ (1987) Modulation of the autologous mixed lymphocyte reaction by β-endorphin. J Neuroimmunol 17(1):1–10

Frohman EM, Frohman TC, Vayuvegula B, Gupta S, van den Noort (1988) Vasoactive intestinal peptide inhibits the expression of the MHC class II antigens on astrocytes. J Neurol Sci 88(1–3): 339–346

Fukata J, Usui T, Naitoh Y, Imura H (1989) Effects of recombinant human interleukin-1-α, β, 2 and 6 on ACTH synthesis and release in the mouse pituitary tumor cell line AtT-20. J Endocrinol 122(1):33–39

Gibbs DM (1986) Vasopressin and oxytocin: hypothalamic regulations of a stress response. Psychoneuroendocrinology 11:131–139

Gilmore W, Weiner LP (1988) β-endorphin enhances interleukin-2 production in murine lymphocytes. J Neuroimmunol 18(2):125–138

Gwosdow AR, Kumar MS, Bode HH (1990) Interleukin-1 stimulation of the hypothalamic-pituitary-adrenal axis. Am J Physiol 250(1,1):E65–70

Hanmann KP, Ruf P, Hopf HC (1988) The inhibitory effects of prednisone, 16-methylen-prednisolone, and ACTH on con-A induced lymphokines (interferon-γ) as measured by the chemiluminesence-activity of blood monocytes. Immunopharmacol Immunotoxicol 19(4):463–478

Harbour DV, Leon S, Keating C, Hughes TK (1990) Thyrotropin modulates B-cell function through specific bioactive receptors. Prog Neuroendocrinimmunol 3:266–276

Harlin CA, Parker CR (1991) Investigation of the effect of interleukin-1-β on steroidogenesis in the human fetal adrenal gland. Steroids 56(2):72–76

Hart R, Dancygier H, Wagner F, Niedermeyer H, Classen M (1988) Substance P modulates lymphokine activities in supernatants of cultured human duodenal mucosa. Immunol Lett 19(2): 133–136

Hart R, Dancygier H, Wagner F, Lersch C, Classen M (1990) Effect of substance P on immunoglobulin and interferon-γ secretion by cultured human duodenal mucosa. Immunol Lett 23(3):199–204

Heijnen CJ, Bevers C, Kavelaars A, Ballieux RE (1986) Effect of α-endorphin on the antigen induced primary antibody response of human blood B cells in vitro. J Immunol 136(1):213–216

Holmgren J, Fryklund J, Larsson H (1989) Gamma interferon mediated down regulation of electrolyte secretion by intestinal epithelial cells: a local immune mechanism? Scand J Immunol 30(4):499–503

Hughes TK (ed) (1992) Interleukins-1 through -8, tumor necrosis factor and interferon-γ. Adv Neuroimmunol 2:1–152

Hughes TK, Smith EM (1989) Corticotropin (ACTH) induction of tumor necrosis factor-α by monocytes. J Biol Regul Homeost Agents 3(4):163–166

Hughes TK, Smith EM, Chin R, Cadet P, Sinisterra J, Leung MK, Shipp MA, Scharrer B, Stefano GB (1990) Interaction of immunoactive monokines (interleukin 1 and tumor necrosis factor) in the bivalve mollusc, Mytilus edulis Proc Natl Acad Sci USA 87:4426–4429

Jaattela M, Carpen O, Stenman UH, Saksela E (1990) Regulation of ACTH-induced steroidogenesis in human fetal adrenals by rTNF-α. Mol Cell Endocrinol 68(2–3):R31–36

Jaattela M, Ilvesmaki V, Voutilainen R, Stenman UH, Saksela E (1991) Tumor necrosis factor as a potent inhibitor of adrenocortropin-induced cortisol production and steroidogenic P450 enzyme gene expression in cultured human fetal adrenal cells. Endocrinology 128(1):623–629

Johnson HM, Torres BA (1985) Regulation of lymphokine production by arginine vasopressin and oxytocin: modulation of lymphocyte function by neurohypophyseal hormones. J Immunol 135(2): 773s–775

Johnson HM, Torres BA (1988) A novel arginine vasopressin binding peptide that blocks arginine vasopressin modulation of immune function. J Immunol 141(7):2420–2423

Johnson HM, Smith EM, Torres BA, Blalock JE (1982a) Neuroendocrine hormone regulation of in vitro antibody production. Proc Natl Acad Sci USA 79:4171–4174

Johnson HM, Farrar WL, Torres BA (1982b) Vasopressin replacement of interleukin-2 requirement in γ-interferon production: lymphokine activity of a neuroendocrine hormone. J Immunol 129(3): 983–986

Johnson HM, Torres BA, Smith EM, Dion LD, Blalock JE (1984) Regulation of lymphokine (α-interferon) production by corticotropin. J Immunol 132:246–250

Karanth S, McCann SM (1991) Anterior pituitary hormone control by interleukin-2. Proc Natl Acad Sci USA 88(7):2961–2964

Kavelaars A, Ballieux RE, Heijnen CJ (1989) The role of interleukin-1 in the corticotropin-releasing factor and arginine vasopressin induced secretion of immunoreactive β-endorphin by human peripheral blood mononuclear cells. J Immunol 142(7):2338–2342

Kavelaars A, Berkenbosch F, Croiset G, Ballieux RE, Heijnen CJ (1990a) Induction of β-endorphin secretion by lymphocytes after subcutaneous administration of corticotropin-releasing factor. Endocrinology 126(2):759–764

Kavelaars A, Ballieux RE, Heijnen CJ (1990b) β-Endorphin secretion by human peripheral blood mononuclear cells: regulation by glucocorticoids. Life Sci 46(17):1233–1240

Kavelaars A, Ballieux RE, Heijnen CJ (1991) Two different signalling pathways for the induction of immunoreactive β-endorphin secretion by human peripheral blood mononuclear cells. Endocrinology 128(2):765–770

Kehrer P, Turnhill D, Dayer JM, Muller AF, Gaillard RC (1988) Human interleukin-1-β and -α, but not recombinant tumor necrosis factor-α stimulate ACTH release from rat anterior pituitary cells in vitro in a prostaglandin E2 and cAMP independent manner. Neuroendocrinology 48(2): 160–166

Kimbala ES, Fischer MC (1988) Potentiation of IL-1 induced BALB/3T3 fibroblast proliferation by neuropeptides. J Immunol 141(12): 4203–4208

Kimball ES, Persico FJ, Vaught JL (1988) Substance P, neurokinin A and neurokinin B induce generation of IL-1 like activity in P388D1 cells. Possible relevance to arthritic disease. J Immunol 141(10):3584–3589

Koff WC, Dunegan MA (1985) Modulation of macrophage mediated tumoricidal activity by neuropeptides and neurohormones. J Immunol 135(1):350–354

Koff WC, Dunegan MA (1986) Neuroendocrine hormones suppress macrophage mediated lysis of herpes simplex virus infected cells. J Immunol 136(2):705–709

Krieger DT (1983) The multiple faces of proopiomelanocortin, a prototype precursor molecule. Clin Res 31:342–353

Krueger TE, Smith LR, Harbour DV, Blalock JE (1989) Thyrotropin: an endogenous regulator of the in vitro immune response. J Immunol 142(3):744–747

Laurentzi MA, Perrson MA, Dalsgaard CJ, Haegerstrand A (1990) The neuropeptide substance P stimulates production of interleukin-1 in human blood monocytes: activated cells are preferentially influenced by the neuropeptide. Scand J Immunol 31(4):529–533

Locher R, Vetter W, Block L (1983) Interactions between 8-L-arginine vasopressin and prostaglandnin E2 in human mononuclear phagocytes. J Clin Invest 71:884–891

Lotz M, Vaughan JH, Carson DA (1988) Effects of neuropeptides on production of inflammatory cytokines by human monocytes. Science 241(4870):1218–1221

Lumpkin MD (1987) The regulation of ACTH secretion by IL-1. Science 238(4826): 452–454

Malarkey WB, Zvara BJ (1989) Interleukin-1-β and other cytokines stimulate adrenocorticotropin release from cultured pituitary cells of patients with Cushing's disease. J Clin Endocrinol Metab 69(1):196–199

Mandler RN, Biddison WE, Mandler R, Serrate SA (1986) β-Endorphin augments the cytolytic activity and interferon production of natural killer cells. J Immunol 136(3):934–939

Martin SB, Tracey KJ (1992) Tumor necrosis factor in neuroimmunology. Adv Neuroimmunol 2: 125–138

Mason J, Van Epps D (1989) Modulation of IL-1, tumor necrosis factor and C5a-mediated murine neutrophil migration by α- melanocyte-stimulating hormone. J Immunol 142(5):1646–1651

McGillis JP, Hall NR, Goldstein AL (1988) Thymosin fraction 5 (TF5) stimulates secretion of adrenocorticotropic hormone (ACTH) from cultured rat pituitaries. Life Sci 42(22):2259–2268

Milenkovic L, Rettori V, Snyder GD, Beutler B, McCann SM (1989) Cachectin alters anterior pituitary hormone release by a direct action in vitro. Proc Natl Acad Sci USA 86(7):2418–2422

Morely JE, Kay N, Allen J, Moon T, Billington CJ (1985) Endorphins, immune function and cancer. Psychopharmacol Bull 21(3):485–488

Naito Y, Fukata J, Shindo K, Ebisui O, Murakami N, Tominaga T, Nakai Y, Mori K, Kasting NW, Imura H (1991) Effects of interleukin on plasma arginine vasopressin and oxytocin levels in conscious, freely moving rats. Biochem Biophys Res Commun 174(3):1189–1195

Nakamura H, Motoyoshi S, Kadokawa T (1988) Anti-inflammatory action of interleukin-1 through the pituitary-adrenal axis in rats. Eur J Pharmacol 151(1):67–73

Natarajan R, Ploszaj S, Horton R, Nadler J (1989) Tumor necrosis factor and interleukin-1 are potent inhibitors of angiotensin-II-induced aldosterone synthesis. Endocrinology 125(6): 3084–3089

Navarra P, Tsagarakis S, Faria MS, Rees LH, Besser GM, Grossman AB (1991) Interleukins 1 and 6 stimulate the release of corticotropin releasing hormone-41 in vitro through the eicosanoid cyclooxygenase pathway. Endocrinology 128(1):37–44

Norman AW, Litwack G (1987) Hormones. Academic Press, Orlando

Oleson DR, Johnson DR (1988) Regulation of human natural cytotoxicity by enkephalins and selective opiate agonists. Brain Behav Immun 2(3):171–186

Opp M, Obai F Jr, Krueger JM (1989) Corticotropin releasing factor attenuates interleukin 1-induced sleep and fever in rabbits. Am J Physiol 257(3 Pt 2):R528–535

Ottaway CA (1987) Selective effects of vasoactive intestinal peptide on the mitogenic response of murine T cells. Immunology 62(2):291–297

Paegelow I, Werner H (1986) Immunomodulation by some oligopeptides. Methods Find Exp Clin Pharmacol 8(2):91–95

Peck R (1987) Neuropeptides modulating macrophage function. Ann NY Acad Sci 496:264–270

Peterson PK, Sharp B, Gekker G, Brumitt C, Keane WF (1987) Opioid mediated suppression of interferon-γ production by cultured peripheral blood mononuclear cells. J Clin Invest 80(3): 824–831

Philip R, Epstein LB (1986) Tumor necrosis factor as immunomodulator and mediator of monocyte cytotoxicity induced by itself, γ interferon and interleukin-1. Nature 323:86–89

Pontzer CH, Griggs ND, Johnson HM (1992) Interleukin-2. Adv Neuroimmunol 2:17–31

Prete P, Levin ER, Pedram A (1986) The in vitro effects of endogenous opiates on natural killer cells, antigen specific cytolytic T-cells and T-cell subsets. Exp Neurol 92(2):349–359

Rettori V, Jurcovicova J, McCann SM (1987) Central action of interleukin-1 in altering the release of TSH, growth hormone and prolactin in the male rat. J Neurosci Res 18(1):179–183

Rettori V, Milenkovic L, Bentler BA, McCann SM (1989) Hypothalamic action of cachectin to alter pituitary hormone release. Brain Res Bull 23:471–475

Rivier C, Vale W, Brown M (1989a) In the rat, interleukin 1-α and -β stimulate adrenocorticotropin and catecholamine release. Endocrinology 125(6):3096–3102

Rivier C, Chizzonite R, Vale W (1989b) In the mouse, the activation of the hypothalamic-pituitary-adrenal axis by lipopolysaccharide (endotoxin) is mediated through interleukin-1. Endocrinology 125(6):2800–2805

Robertson BA, Gahring LC, Daynes RA (1986) Neuropeptide regulation of interleukin-1 activities. Capacity of α-melanocyte stimulating hormone to inhibit interleukin-1-inducible responses in vivo and in vitro exhibits target cell selectivity. Inflammation 10(4):371–385

Rossi NF, Schrier RW (1986) Role of arginine vasopressin in regulation of systemic arterial pressure. Annu Rev Med 37:13–20

Sawyer WH (1961) Neurohypophyseal hormones. Pharmacol Rev 13:225–277

Schettini G, Florio T, Meucci O, Landolfi E, Grimaldi M, Lombardi G, Scala G, Leong D (1990) Interleukin-1-β modulation of prolactin secretion from rat anterior pituitary cells: involvement of adenylate cyclase activity and calcium mobilization. Endocrinology 126(3):1435–1441

Schiogolev SA, Goetzl EJ, Urba WJ, Longo DL (1989) Appearance of neuropeptides in ascitic fluid after peritoneal therapy with interleukin-2 and lymphokine activated killer cells for intra-abdominal therapy. J Clin Immunol 9(2):169–173

Sharp BM, Matta SO, Peterson PK, Newton R, Chao C, Mcallen K (1989) Tumor necrosis factor-α is a potent ACTH secretagogue: comparison to interleukin-1-β. Endocrinology 124(6): 3131–3133

Smith EM (1991) Hormonal activities of cytokines. Prog Allergy (in press)

Smith EM, Blalock JE (1981) Human lymphocyte production of ACTH and endorphin-like substances: association with leucocyte interferon. Proc Natl Acad Sci USA 78:7530–7534

Smith LR, Brown SL, Blalock JE (1989) Interleukin-2 induction of ACTH secretion: presence of an interleukin-2 receptor α-chain-like molecule on pituitary cells. J Neuroimmunol 21(2–3):249–254

Spangelo BL, Judd AM, Isakson PC, MacLeod RM (1991) Interleukin-1 stimulates interleukin-6 release from rat anterior pituitary cells in vitro. Endocrinology 128(6):2685–2692

Stefano GB (1989) Role of opioid neuropeptides in immunoregulation. Prog Neurobiol 33:149–159

Stefano GB, Smith EM, Hughes TK (1991) Opioid induction of immunoreactive IL-1 in Mytilus edulis and human immunocytes: an IL-1 like substance in invertebrate neural tissue. J Neuroimmunol 32:29–34

Suda T, Tozawa F, Ushiyama T, Sumitomo T, Yamada M, Demura H (1990) Interleukin-1 stimulates corticotropin-releasing factor gene expression in rat hypothalamus. Endocrinology 126(2): 1223–1228

Taverne J, Rayner DC, Van Der Meide PH, Lydyard PM, Bidey SP (1987) Cytotoxicity of tumor necrosis factor for thyroid epithelial cells and its regulation by interferon-γ. Eur J Immunol 17(12); 1855–1858

Tepperman J (1980) Metabolic and endocrine physiology. Year Book Medical Publishers. Chicago, 73

Todd I, Pujol-Borrel R, Hammond LJ, McNally JM, Feldmann M, Bottazzo GF (1987a) Enhancement of thyroid class II expression by thyroid stimulating hormone. Clin Exp Immunol 69(3):524–531

Todd I, Pujo-Borrell R, Belfore A, Bottazzo F (1987b) Thyrocyte class II expression and regulation in relation to thyroid autoimmunity. Acta Endocrinol (copenh) (suppl) 281:27–34

Todd I, Hammond LJ, James RF, Feldmann M, Bottazzo GF (1990) Epidermal growth factor and transforming growth α suppress HLA class II induction in human thyroid epithelial cells. Immunology 69(1):91–96

Tominaga T, Fukata J, Naito Y, Usui T, Murakami N, Fukushima M, Nakai Y, Hirai Y, Imura H (1991) Prostaglandin-dependent in vitro stimulation of adrenocortical steroidogenesis by interleukins. Endocrinology 128(1):526–531

Torres BA, HM Johnson (1988) Arginine vasopressin (AVP) replacement of helper cell requirement in IFN-γ production. Evidence for a noval AVP receptor on mouse lymphocytes. J Immunol 140(7):2179–2183

Torres-Aleman I, Barasoain I, Borrell J, Guaza C (1988) Immune activation and psychoneurogenic stress modulate corticosterone-releasing effects of lymphokines and ACTH. Am J Physiol 255(5,2): R839–845

Uehara A, Gottschall PE, Dahl RR, Arimura A (1987a) Interleukin-1 stimulates ACTH release by an indirect action which requires endogenous corticotropin releasing factor. Endocrinology 121(4):1580–1582

Uehara A, Gottschall PE, Dahl RR, Arimura A (1987b) Stimulation of ACTH release by human interleukin-1-β, but not by human interleukin-1-α, in conscious, freely-moving rats. Biochem Biophys Res Commun 146(3):1286–1290

Uehara A, Gillis S, Arimura A (1987c) Effects of interleukin-1 on hormone release from normal rat pituitary cells in culture. Neuroendocrinology 45(5):343–347

Vankelecom H, Billiau A (1992) Interferon-γ in neuroimmunology and endocrinology. Adv Neuroimmunol 2:139–161

Vankelecom H, Carmeleit P, Heremans H, Van Damme J, Dijkmans R, Billiau A, Denef C (1990) Interferon-γ inhibits stimulated adrenocorticotropin, prolactin, and growth hormone secretion in normal rat anterior pituitary cell cultures. Endocrinology 126(6):2919–2926

Van-den-Bergh P, Rozing J, Nagelkerken L (1991) Two opposing modes of action of β endorphin on lymphocyte function. Immunology 72(4):537–543

Wagner F, Fink R, Hart R, Dancygier H (1987) Substance P enhances interferon-γ production by human peripheral blood mononuclear cells. Regul Pept 19(5–6):355–364

Weidenfield J, Abramsky O, Ovadia H (1989) Evidence for the involvement of the central adrenergic system in interleukin-1 induced adrenocortical response. Neuropharmacology 28(12):1411–1414

Weigent DA, Blalock JE (1987) Interactions between the neuroendocrine and immune systems: common hormones and receptors. Immunol Rev 100:79–108

Weiss JM, Sundar SK, Cierpal MA, Ritchie JC (1991) Effects of interleukin-1 infused into the brain are antagonized by α-MSH in a dose-dependent manner. Eur J Pharmacol 192(1):177–179

Woloski BMRNJ, Smith EM, Meyer WJ III, Fuller GM, Blalock JE (1985) Corticotropin releasing activity of monokines. Science 230:1035–1037

Zadina JE, Banks WA, Kastin AJ (1986) Central nervous system effects of peptides, 1980–1985: a cross listing of peptides and their central actions form the first six years of jorunal. Peptides 7(3):497–537

Stress and Immunity

J. A. Moynihan[1], N. Cohen[2], and R. Ader[1]

Introduction

For many years immunologists have considered an immune response to be a direct consequence of, and solely determined by, antigenic stimulation of an autonomous immune system. In the past decade, however, we have come to realize that the immune system is regulated by the central nervous system either directly, or by way of the neuroendocrine axis, i.e., the hypothalamic-hypophysial system, or the autonomic nervous system (Ader et al. 1990). The realization that the central nervous system has immunomodulatory potential is based on many different lines of evidence. For example, primary and secondary lymphoid organs are innervated by the sympathetic nervous system (Felten and Felten 1991), and lymphoid cells express cell-surface receptors for β-adrenergic transmitters, as well as receptors for a host of neurally and neuroendocrinologically active peptides (Blalock 1988; Weigent and Blalock, this volume). A large number of hormones and transmitters have been shown to exert immunomodulatory effects both in vivo and in vitro (see Khansari et al. 1990). These include:

Glucocorticoids (Munck and Guyre 1991)
Opioids – endorphins and enkephalins (Shavit 1991; Heijen et al. 1991)
Catecholamines – dopamine, epinephrine, norepinephrine (Madden and Livnat 1991)
Acetylcholine (Coffey and Hadden 1985)
Benzodiazepines (Petitto et al. 1989)
Gonadal hormones – testosterone, estrogen, progesterone (McCruden and Stimson 1991)
Adrenocorticotropin (Heijen et al. 1991)
Growth hormone (Ader et al. 1990; Kelley 1991)
Prolactin (Bernton et al. 1991)
Vasoactive intestinal peptide (Ottaway 1991)
Somatostatin (Stanisz et al. 1986)
Substance P (McGillis et al. 1991)
Thymic hormones – thymopoetin, thymopentin (Hall et al. 1991)

[1] Department of Psychiatry, University of Rochester Medical Center, 601, Elmwood Avenue, Rochester, NY 14642, USA
[2] Department of Microbiology and Immunology, University of Rochester Medical Center, 601, Elwood Avenue, Rochester, NY 14642, USA

Scharrer et al. (Eds.)
Neuropeptides and Immunoregulation

Thyroid hormones – thyrotropin, thyrotropin-releasing hormone (Carr and Blalock 1991)
Melatonin (Maestroni and Conti 1991)
Vasopressin (Johnson and Torres 1985)
Oxytocin (Johnson and Torres 1985)

Learning, as exemplified by classical conditioning, can enhance (Gorczynski 1991) or depress (Ader and Cohen 1991) immune responses. These effects are mediated largely, but not exclusively, by the hypothalamic-hypophysial-adrenal axis. Therefore, experiments with various types of stress are required to provide information on the roles played by neuropeptides in concert with various other signal molecules involved in neuroimmunomodulation.

Stress, as defined by the scientist and physician Selye (1950), is any deviation from homeostasis, the normal resting condition. He wrote that, "any change affecting a living organism is a stressor, as it elicits some efforts to resist and, hence, at least mild manifestations of an alarm reaction." It is now accepted that stressor administration causes complex neurological and neurochemical changes as the host attempts to adapt to that stressor. These neural and endocrine changes are important in regulating many physiological processes (e.g., those involved in maintaining blood pressure or body temperature), including those that can regulate immune function. These immunomodulatory changes can, in turn, modify the host response to pathogens and, presumably, its health status.

The literature dealing with the effects of stress on immunity documents immune alterations in a variety of species that have been subjected to different stresses applied at different times in relation to measurements of different immunological outcomes. Some of these stressors are physical (e.g., electric footshock) and others are psychosocial (e.g., infant–mother separation). There is no evidence to indicate that all these stressors evoke the same series or pattern of neurochemical changes in the experimental subject.

Studies involving different stresssors have revealed changes in specific immune functions as well as nonspecific components of the defense systems of stressed, compared with putatively nonstressed, animals. Other studies have examined stress-associated changes in the response to tumors or microbial pathogens without examining alterations in immune function per se.

This chapter reviews stress-induced changes in specific humoral and cell-mediated immunity, natural killer (NK) cell activity, mitogen-induced lymphocyte proliferation, and numbers of lymphocytes in different subsets. As described below, the use of each of these parameters has its associated strengths and weaknesses in terms of generality and applicability to understanding the effects of stress on immunity in the "real world." For example, mitogen-induced proliferation of lymphocytes does not reflect specific immune function per se. Whereas lipopolysaccharide (LPS) can activate proliferation of approximately 20% of B-lymphocytes from a nonimmune animal, and LPS plus dextran sulfate can drive proliferation of 80% of B-cells in the absence of T-cells and macrophages, less than 1% of the B-cells from a deliberately immunized animal are triggered by antigen (Feldbush et al. 1986). Thus, a stress-associated change in mitogen responsiveness may not reflect actual changes in an animal's ability to respond to antigen in an immunologically specific fashion. Alternatively, stress-induced changes in mitogenesis may be an indicator of a change in the number of lymphocytes in a particular lymphoid compartment, differences in the availability of cytokines (or their receptors) that play a role in mitogenesis, and/or an altered physiological state of the responding lymphocyte itself.

Many studies detailing stress-induced immune modulation, including some studies that focus on antigen-specific responses, rely on in vitro assays of cellular function. These studies may be limited in terms of the lymphoid compartment from which cells are harvested. They also do not provide the neuroendocrine milieu in which a stress response normally occurs. That is, removing T- and B-lymphocytes or NK cells from both the whole organism and the splenic or lymph node architecture may mask changes that are actually occurring in different lymphoid compartments in the animal (Rabin et al. 1990).

Although numerous studies have demonstrated stress-associated changes in activity and/or numbers of NK cells in humans and experimental animals, the role played by these large granular lymphocytes in host resistance to viral infections or tumorigenesis is still not entirely clear.

As a final caveat, it should be noted that several of the studies that have looked for changes in immune function have yielded equivocal results. The failure to demonstrate clear-cut stress-induced changes in specific immunity may be related to the use of a so-called immunologically optimal concentration of antigen (i.e., one that elicits maximal immune responses) that masks subtle regulatory effects of stress, rather than a lesser amount of antigen that more closely approximates antigen exposure in a natural setting (Moynihan et al. 1989).

Despite these caveats concerning limitations of immune measures, it is still apparent that stressor application can alter immune function. This chapter is organized according to the diversity of psychosocial and physical stress models that have provided evidence of stress-induced immunomodulation in animals. Owing to space restrictions, the review is illustrative rather than exhaustive (for additional information, see reviews by Sklar and Anisman 1981; Ader and Cohen 1985; Glaser et al. 1987; Rabin et al. 1989; Dantzer and Kelley 1989; Cohen and Williamson 1991; Moynihan and Cohen 1990; Kemeny et al. 1991).

Aggression/Social Conflict

To examine the effects of aggressive encounters on immunity, animals are exposed to other animals, and a dominance hierarchy is established as determined either by submissive and dominant posturings or by actual numbers of fights that end in defeat of one member of the pair. Immune responsiveness is measured in the established dominant and submissive animals. In a number of instances, interpretation of these results is complicated by the possibility that the wounding of animals might be associated with immune changes. As is the case with other stress paradigms, different strains and species of rodents have been examined, different antigens have been used, and the stressor has been applied at different times in relation to the immune outcome measure. Beden and Brain (1982, 1984) reported that male mice that were defeated by a trained "attacker mouse" more than three times had significantly reduced primary, but unaffected secondary, anti-sheep red blood cell (SRBC) antibody titers. Ito et al. (1983) immunized male rats with dinitrophenyl-*Ascaris* following three attack sessions and observed no effect on a primary IgE antibody response. When the attacks preceded secondary immunization, however, the secondary antibody response was suppressed. Fleshner et al. (1989) introduced male rats successively into each of five aggressive colonies during two sessions. The "intruder" rats subsequently produced a significantly reduced primary IgG anti-keyhole limpet hemocyanin (KLH) antibody response.

Hardy et al. (1990) determined that submissive male mice had lower T-cell proliferative responses to concanavalin A (Con A) and phytohemagglutinin (PHA) and lower production of interleukin 2/4 (IL-2/4) than either dominant mice, "not-fought" control mice, or mice that merely witnessed aggressive encounters. No significant group differences were found in the splenic NK response of any of these animals. The effects of social conflict on mitogen-induced proliferation and nonspecific cytotoxicity against the tumor target YAC-1 (cytotoxicity due to NK-like cells) have also been examined in the teleost fish *Tilapia* (Ghoneum et al. 1988). Submissive fish had lower responses to Con A, PHA, and LPS, and depressed cytotoxic responses compared to fish that were either dominant or those that were "not fought". Further, the numbers of mononuclear cells were decreased, and polymorphonuclear leukocytes were increased in the submissive animals following social conflict (Peters and Schwarzer 1985; Ghoneum et al. 1988). In a related series of experiments (Faisal et al. 1989), sera from submissive, dominant, or control fish were added to mitogen-treated cultures of pronephric leukocytes from fish in each of the three groups. Sera from submissive fish depressed the mitogen response of the control and dominant fish to T-cell mitogens, but not to LPS. The suppressive effect of this serum was largely abolished, however, when the donor submissive animals were injected with naltrexone prior to social conflict. In contrast, naltrexone treatment did not restore the suppressed levels of cytotoxicity in leukocyte cultures from submissive animals, nor did it fully restore the levels of Con A and PHA responsiveness in leukocytes from these animals. Thus, opioid peptides appear to play a role in some, but certainly not all, aspects of the alteration of immune responses following social conflict in fish.

Infant–Mother Separation

Another paradigm used to study the effects of stress on antibody production involves infant–mother separation. Michaut et al. (1980) removed mothers from litters of mice for 4–8 h/day during the first 2 weeks of life and observed reduced serum antibody titers and plaque-forming cell (PFC) responses to SRBC in the offspring following immunization at 8 weeks of age. Coe et al. (1987) reported that infant squirrel monkeys had a reduced antibody response to a bacteriophage when they were separated from their mothers and maintained alone in an unfamiliar environment. Monkeys that had the lowest antibody titers also had the highest levels of plasma cortisol and sustained these high levels for the longest period of time.

Infant separation need not always be immunosuppressive. For example, Solomon et al. (1968) placed individual rat pups from group-housed cages in boxes for 3 min/day from birth to weaning and measured a primary and secondary antibody response to flagellin at 9 and 13 weeks of age. The rat pups that had been removed from the nesting cages actually had higher primary and secondary responses than unmanipulated controls.

Handling

Another psychosocial manipulation that has immunomodulatory effects is the handling of experimental animals. We have demonstrated that holding adult mice gently in the palm of the hand for 2 min daily for 2 weeks prior to immunization reduces their IgG primary antibody response to the T-cell dependent protein antigen KLH (Moynihan et al. 1989, 1990a). Splenocytes from handled mice have a lower proliferative response to the T-cell mitogen Con A but not to the B-cell mitogen LPS relative to unhandled animals. Total numbers of spleen cells, cells in various lymphocyte subsets, and the NK response were unaffected by this handling protocol. We have also demonstrated that handling adult mice for 2 weeks results in an increase in pulmonary metastases following intravenous injection of syngeneic line 1 tumor cells (Brenner et al. 1990); whether this is immunologically mediated remains to be determined.

Lown and Dutka (1987) found no evidence of altered Con A reactivity in splenocytes from mice that were moved to a different cage for 10 min daily from weaning until day 60 of age. However, adult mice that were manipulated in this fashion from birth until weaning had an enhanced mitogen response relative to unmanipulated controls. The age at which an animal is handled is an important factor in the modulation of an immune response.

Early handling experiences have also been shown to alter antibody responses. For example, neonatal handling suppressed the antibody response of adult C57BL/10J mice but not BALB/cJ mice (Raymond et al. 1986). Although neonatal handling has also been reported to increase susceptibility to transplanted tumors (Newton et al. 1962; Ader and Friedman 1965), the role of the immune system in this altered susceptibility is unknown.

Aquaculture of fish often requires handling and transport of the animals, procedures that have been associated with increased morbidity and mortality due to bacterially and virallly mediated diseases (Wedemeyer 1970). Ellsaesser and Clem (1986) and Bly et al. (1990) observed that "transport stress" of channel catfish was associated with a dramatic reduction in the primary PFC response to the T-cell-dependent antigen KLH and the T-cell independent antigen LPS, and with decreases in numbers of mononuclear cells. Ellsaesser and Clem (1986) also noted a depressed response to Con A and LPS in lymphocytes from transported catfish 18 h after they had been returned to their home tanks. The depressed mitogen responses recovered in 3–4 weeks, sometimes exceeding baseline values. Further observations by the same investigators (Ellsaesser and Clem 1987) and by Tripp et al. (1987) suggest a role for plasma cortisol in this immunosuppression. That is, injecting non-transported fish with doses of cortisol equivalent to the levels found in transported fish caused a similar reduction in mitogen responses.

Differential Housing

The manner in which animals are housed and alterations in their housing conditions can influence immunological reactivity. Vessey (1964) found that individually housed male mice had higher antibody responses to bovine serum than did individually housed mice that were transferred to a group-housing situation for 4 h/day. Rabin et al. (1987) and Rabin and Salvin (1987) examined the effects of group versus individual housing on a number of immunological responses in male and female C3H and male C57/BL6J mice. Male C3H mice that were individually housed for 10–14 days displayed increased resistance to infection with *Candida albicans* compared to group-housed mice. In addition, the proliferative response of splenocytes to Con A, in vitro IL-2/4 synthesis, and the PFC response to SRBC were greater in individually-housed animals. After 3 weeks of individual housing, however, significant differences were no longer seen. It is noteworthy that differential housing did not influence any of these immune responses in female C3H or male C57BL/6J mice.

In a study by Edwards et al. (1980), male mice were housed individually from weaning until 16 weeks of age, at which time they were immunized with bovine serum albumin (BSA) and then placed into cages with "socialized" females. Seven days later, mice were reimmunized, and half of the males were returned to individual cages and half remained in the social environment. Mice that were exposed to group-housing and then returned to isolation had a significantly depressed anti-BSA antibody titer compared to the other half of the males.

Ghoneum et al. (1987) examined the effects of group versus individual housing on NK cell function in young (3-month) or "old" (12-month) rats. NK cell activity was depressed in individually-housed aged rats compared to group-housed aged rats. Interestingly, no differences were observed in the young rats.

In one series of experiments, Solomon (1969) compared the effects of three different stressors (differential housing, footshock, and REM sleep deprivation) on the primary and secondary anti-flagellin antibody responses in male Fisher rats. Differential housing (i.e., a change from 2 to 5 or 6 per cage) resulted in significantly depressed primary and secondary antibody responses. Footshock, however, resulted in no changes in antibody responsiveness, and sleep deprivation depressed the primary but not the secondary antibody response. These important studies clearly point out that in a single laboratory, different stressors can have different qualitative and perhaps even quantitative effects on a single parameter of immunity.

Restraint

In the first of an elegant series of studies, Okimura and Nigo (1986) evaluated several immune responses in mice that were restrained for 12 h/day on 2 consecutive days. Restraint depressed the PFC and serum antibody response to SRBC when it was administered before, but not after, immunization. Injection of the antianxiolytic drug diazepam (a benzodiazepine) significantly abrogated the effect of restraint on the anti-SRBC PFC response. Further, although spleen cell numbers were decreased in restrained mice, there was no difference in relative percentages of T- or B-cells. Finally, the PFC responses to haptens conjugated to the T-cell independent carriers Ficoll and LPS were not suppressed by restraint before immunization. Subsequently, Okimura et al. (1986a) reported that the anti-TNP Ficoll response was unaffected by restraint, and the LPS response was actually enhanced by restraint stressor administration. These observations led the investigators to hypothesize that T-cell function is impaired by restraint, but that B-cell activity is not negatively influenced by the treatment. Whether stressors differentially affect the response to thymus-independent (TI) antigens that are type 1 (such as LPS), which activate a relatively more immature population of B-cells than TI type 2 antigens (such as Ficoll) remains to be determined. Okimura et al. (1986b) also found that restraint decreases macrophage phagocytosis and NK cell cytotoxicity and depresses the delayed-type hypersensitivity (DTH) response to SRBC.

Adrenalectomy blocks both the restraint-induced suppression of the response to the T-dependent antigen SRBC and the enhancement of the response to LPS (Okimura et al. 1986c). Phenoxybenzamine or 6-hydroxydopamine pretreatment prevented the depression of the response to SRBC, but did not affect the enhanced response to LPS. Thus, the results of these experiments suggest that restraint could depress T-cell function via release of adrenal corticosteroids and activation of the sympathetic nervous system. However, B-cell function was unaffected in this paradigm by sympathetic activation.

Blecha et al. (1982a,b) noted a depressed DTH response to SRBC in mice that were restrained for 2.5 h before either primary immunization or challenge with SRBC. In contrast, contact sensitivity to dinitrofluorobenzene was enhanced in restrained animals. These investigators further determined that adrenalectomy or metapyrone treatment abolishes the stressor-induced suppression of the DTH response but does not affect the observed enhancement of the contact sensitivity response, indicating that different effector functions are regulated by different neuroendocrine pathways.

Steplewski et al. (1985; Steplewski and Vogel 1986) found that restraining rats for 3 h/day for 11–12 successive days results in a decreased absolute number (but unaffected ratio) of CD4 and CD8 positive peripheral blood T-cells. NK cell activity was unaffected by this treatment. In some experiments rats were allowed to recover from the restraint for an additional 12 days and were then injected with a mammary adenocarcinoma. Rats that had been stressed and allowed to recover had decreased tumor growth compared to animals that had not recovered.

Rotation

Mice were rotated at 100 rpm for a total of five cycles (10 min of rotation followed by 50 min of rest) daily for either 3 or 4 days (Esterling and Rabin 1987). The PFC response to SRBC was depressed when rotation was begun 24 h after (3 days of rotation) but not when it was initiated on the same day as (4 days of rotation) immunization; however, the numbers of splenic Ly-1^+ and Ly-2^+ T-cells were depressed in both groups. Interestingly, adrenalectomy prior to rotation did not alter the depression of the PFC response. Further, adrenalectomized mice recovered their numbers of Ly-1^+ T-cells regardless of the number of rotation sessions to which they had been subjected. The numbers of Ly-2^+ cells returned to normal only in those mice that were rotated for a total of four sessions. These data indicate that there is a complex interaction between the amount or timing of stressor application, changes in neuroendocrine function, and immune responsiveness.

Electric Shock
Predictability, Control, and Conditioning

Electric shock has been the most commonly used stimulus for studying stress effects on immune function, since a number of interacting variables can be manipulated (e.g., number and length of shock sessions, varying intensity of shock, predictable versus unpredictable onset, and controllability).

Keller et al. (1981, 1984) examined the effects of low-versus high-intensity, unpredictable tailshock of rats on numbers of circulating lymphocytes and the response to PHA in rats. Rats were restrained and shocked for a total of 22 h. The shock groups received 2–5 shocks at variable times but averaging one per minute. For the low-intensity shock group, the current intensity was initially 0.8 mA and was increased over time to 1.2 mA. The high-intensity shock group received 1.6–3.0 mA. A whole blood assay for measuring PHA-induced proliferation revealed highly significant group differences. Specifically, the shock groups had significantly lower mitogen responses than either home-cage and apparatus control groups, and those of the low-intensity shock group were higher than those of the high-intensity shock group. There was a marked lymphocytopenia in both of the shock groups, but there were no differences in the percentage of peripheral blood T-cells. Interestingly, when the mitogen assay was performed with a constant number of isolated lymphocytes, the difference between the two shock groups was obscured, although both groups still differed from both the apparatus and home-cage control groups. Thus, the intensity of shock is a factor in the modulation of the immune response, but its effects may be obscured by the culture conditions chosen.

In a subsequent series of experiments, Keller et al. (1983) examined the effects of adrenalectomy on the PHA responses of lymphocytes from low- and high-intensity shocked rats. In the whole blood assay and with isolated lymphocytes, adrenalectomy did not abrogate the suppression of the PHA response in shocked animals. The observed lymphocytopenia, however, was adrenal dependent. In addition, Keller et al. (1988) determined that hypophysectomy results in loss of some stress-induced change in immune response (numbers of leukocytes) while resulting in increased suppression of the peripheral blood mitogen response.

Laudenslager et al. (1988) exposed rats to unpredictable and inescapable tailshock during one or three daily sessions/week for 2 consecutive weeks. Prior to the onset of any shock sessions, rats were immunized with KLH and received a second immunization 1 week later. The immunizations were carried out during either the light or dark phase of the rats' light cycle. Eight weeks following the initial immunization rats were given a third injection of KLH. Regardless of the conditions of tailshock (one versus three daily sessions), shocked rats had depressed primary and secondary IgG anti-KLH antibody responses. There was no interaction between immunization, light cycle, and shock.

The effects of stressors on immune function may be rather subtle and thus perhaps masked by the use of "optimal" or suprathreshold concentrations of antigen to elicit humoral responses. Optimal refers to doses of antigen that elicit robust primary and secondary antibody responses and are doses that might have no relevance to amounts of antigen encountered in nature. Therefore, we (Moynihan et al. 1990b) examined the effects of footshock stress administered to mice at the time of priming with a low dose of KLH on the secondary antibody response to KLH. The immunizing doses (0.2–1.0 μg) did not elicit detectable primary responses as measured by an enzyme-linked immunoassay. In the first set of experiments, signalled footshock was administered 7 days before and 7 days after primary immunization. A depressed secondary antibody response in the footshocked mice was observed when the priming concentration of antigen was 1 μg and the secondary immunization was 1 μg, but not 5 μg, of KLH. In further studies it was determined that a single session, but not three or seven sessions, of footshock beginning 24 h after priming results in a depressed IgG anti-KLH antibody response. Thus, the dose of antigen used to elicit an antibody response, as well as the timing of the stressor administration, are factors in this model of stress-induced immune modulation.

Laudenslager et al. (1983) compared the effects of escapable versus inescapable tailshock on the lymphocyte response to PHA and Con A. Home-cage and apparatus control rats were included. No differences were found in peripheral blood white cell counts among the groups. Inescapable, but not escapable, shock was associated with a depression in the Con A and PHA responses. Maier and Laudenslager (1988), however, have reported their inability to reproduce this difference.

Mormede et al. (1988) studied the effects of prediction and control of electric shock on immune function in rats. Rats received signalled or nonsignalled inescapable shock during two 30-min daily sessions. At the end of the second shock session plasma corticosterone was significantly elevated in both shock groups compared to control rats. The Con A response of the unsignalled shock group was decreased compared to both the predictable shock and control groups. In a second experiment, rats were trained to avoid shock in a shuttlebox apparatus. The avoidance group had a yoked control associated with it. These animals received the same amount of shock as the avoidance group but had no means to control shock. An apparatus control was included. Rats were given ten daily shock sessions, and in some groups were immunized with SRBC following the fifth avoidance session. After the tenth session lymphocyte proliferative responses, serum anti-SRBC antibody titers, plasma corticosterone, and prolactin levels were measured. The anti-SRBC antibody response of the avoidance group was depressed compared to both control and yoked rats. No effect of shock on the response to Con A or pokeweed mitogen was observed in either the avoidance or yoked groups compared to control rats, but the response to PHA was suppressed in the yoked group at the highest concentration of mitogen. Plasma corticosterone and prolactin levels were significantly increased in both avoidance and yoked groups compared to control animals. These experiments indicate, again, that the effects of stress on different immune parameters may differ, and that some of these effects are independent of adrenocortical steroids, since both the avoidance and predictable shock groups had increased glucocorticoid levels but no suppression of mitogen responses.

Zalcman et al. (1988) immunized mice with SRBC and subjected them to a single footshock session 0, 24, 48, 72, or 95 h after immunization. Both the number of PFCs and that of serum antibody titers sampled 96 h after immunization were depressed only in the mice that were subjected to footshock 72 h after immunization. This suggests that there is a critical period during which shock-associated immune changes can result in an altered antibody response. Using a single shock session 72 h after immunization, these investigators further demonstrated that mice that were allowed to escape shock had depressed PFC responses compared to nonshocked controls. The mice that could control shock by escaping also did not differ in their responses from yoked animals, those that experienced the same amount of shock but did not have the ability to control the shock. Thus, the ability to escape or control shock did not alter the effects of shock on the PFC response to SRBC.

In subsequent experiments, Zalcman et al. (1989) used their footshock paradigm to demonstrate alterations in the PFC and serum antibody responses to SRBC following exposure to stressor-related cues. Mice were exposed to the footshock 2 weeks before immunization with SRBC. Three days after immunization, mice were placed in the shock boxes but were not shocked. Rather, they were merely picked up by the tail and returned to their home cages or left unmanipulated in the home cage. Mice that were reexposed to the shock boxes but not shocked had suppressed antibody responses compared to the other groups. When mice were initially shocked immediately following immunization and then reexposed to the shock boxes, an enhanced antibody response was observed relative to the home cage controls. These data suggest the possibility of conditioned stress effects in the modulation of humoral immunity. They also reemphasize the point that the effect of stress on the immune response to antigen is dependent upon the time of stressor application.

Lysle et al. (1987) found that signalled footshock, given 8 or 16 times in a single shock session, suppresses the Con A response of both splenic and peripheral blood lymphocytes in rats. They also demonstrated (Lysle et al. 1988) that this stress-associated depression could be conditioned when rats were exposed to a single session of signalled (a light plus clicking sound) footshock, allowed to recover for 6 days, and then reexposed to the conditioned stimulus (CS, the light and clicking sound) alone. The depression of the mitogen response could be attenuated by either preexposure to the CS or by extinction (unreinforced CS presentations). Thus, the depressed mitogen response could be elicited by stressor-associated cues in the absence of physical footshock. Whether the neuroendocrine mechanisms underlying the depression associated with the physical stimulus of footshock are the same as those that are associated with CS-induced suppression remains to be determined.

Lysle et al. (1987) found that the Con A response of peripheral blood lymphocytes remains depressed when rats are subjected to three or five daily footshock sessions (each composed of 8 or 16 footshocks). The proliferative response of splenic lymphocytes, however, recovered to control levels by five sessions. It was hypothesized that habituation to the footshock had occurred, and that habituation is more rapid in the spleen than in peripheral blood. (For a discussion of habituation and stress see a review by Moynihan et al. 1991). A recent study by Rabin et al. (1990) showed that the depression of the mitogen response in peripheral blood lymphocytes of rats is absent in adrenalectomized animals, but that the depression in the splenic mitogen response is adrenal independent. Evidently, different lymphoid compartments respond differently to stressors, and may be differentially regulated by different neuroendocrine pathways.

Although the literature has concentrated on the role of corticosteroids in stress-induced immune modulation, many other neuroendocrine changes that occur in response to stressors are important for regulating changes in immune function. In fact, as has been pointed out in this review, not all stress-induced immune changes are adrenal dependent (e.g., Keller et al. 1983). Using a footshock model, Shavit et al. (1986, 1991) demonstrated a role of opioids in the stress-induced suppression of NK cell cytotoxicity. Exposure of rats to prolonged intermittent footshock for varying numbers of days resulted in opioid analgesia. This footshock paradigm, as opposed to continuously applied footshock (which does not induce opioid analgesia), resulted in a significant suppression of the NK cells cytotoxic response to the YAC-1 tumor cell target. This suppression was blocked by administration of the opioid antagonist naltrexone and was mimicked by morphine administration. It should be noted that opioids are not always involved in stress-induced suppression of NK cell cytotoxicity (Ben-Eliyahu et al. 1990).

Using the footshock paradigm (16 shocks for 1 or 5 sessions) described above (Lysle et al. 1987), Cunnick et al. (1988) also demonstrated a depression of splenic NK cell cytotoxicity against YAC-1 cells. Although the suppressed mitogen response of spleen cells recovered following five shock sessions, the NK cell function of these cells remained suppressed. This suppression of NK cell function was abolished by prior treatment with naltrexone, but this treatment did not affect suppression of the mitogen response. Diazepam, which binds to the benzodiazepine receptor and is used clinically in the treatment of anxiety, did not affect the suppression of either the mitogen or NK cell response. Again, these data collectively indicate that stressor application results in altered neurochemical pathways that differentially affect different lymphoid compartments and different immune functions in a given compartment.

As mentioned above, Solomon (1969) described the effects of footshock on the primary and secondary anti-flagellin antibody responses in rats. Footshock was administered beginning 1 week prior to primary immunization and was continued on a daily basis throughout the experiment. The conditions were signalled shock administered randomly five times/h for 8–10 h/day with increasing amperage over time to reduce the chance of habituation. This treatment did not alter the antibody response to the concentration of antigen administered.

Chronic Stressor Administration

Most of the available literature addresses the effects of short-term or acute stress on immune functions; few studies have examined differences in immune responses as a function of the duration of exposure to a stressor or attempted to define the differences between acute and chronic stress presentation. Critical periods for stressor administration and habituation following a brief number of stressor applications have been reported. One such study that demonstrated such a dynamic response to daily stressor application over approximately a 6-week period is that of Monjan and Collector (1977). Mice were exposed to 100 dB broad-band noise for 1–3 h daily. At various times mice were killed, and their splenic mitogen response to Con A and LPS was assayed. In some cases mice were immunized 9 days before killing with P815 tumor targets, and the ability of their spleen cells to lyse P815 cells in vitro was assayed. Plasma cortisol measurements were also made. Biphasic curves were generated for the responsiveness to mitogens and the ability to lyse tumor target cells. Initially these responses were depressed (1–10 days). At approximately 20 days the immune measures returned to baseline and were subsequently enhanced compared to prestimulation levels. The mitogen responses returned to baseline at approximately 40 days. Plasma corticosterone levels were elevated until about 15 days. Mice maintained a baseline steroid level for the remainder of the measurements. These data conform to the kinetics of the general-adaptation syndrome of Selye (1950), in which the initial resistance (response) of the host to a stressor is depressed, followed by recovery, and then enhanced resistance for some period of time. According to Selye, the stage of adaptation would be followed by "exhaustion," a period in which resistance to stress declines, and ultimately death occurs. The final stage of exhaustion and death might require months or years of stressor application to occur.

Neuroendocrine Mechanisms of Stress-Induced Immunomodulation

Current information on stress-induced changes in immunoregulation indicates that different stressors may elicit different humoral as well as cell-mediated immune responses. In most cases the levels of various immunoactive messenger substances are altered, but conclusions drawn from such experimental results regarding the roles of the substances in immunomodulation are largely inferential.

Not all of the stress-induced phenomena investigated have been found to involve the hypothalmic-hypophysial-adrenal axis. Increased levels of glucocorticoids produced in response to stressor administration have been correlated with alterations of some immune functions (Blecha et al. 1982b; Okimura et al. 1986c; Coe et al. 1987; Rabin et al. 1990). However, it is quite clear that stress-induced modulation of immune responses can occur in adrenalectomized or hypopysectomized animals (Blecha et al. 1982b; Esterling and Rabin 1987; Keller et al. 1983, 1988; Rabin et al. 1990), and that altered immune function may occur in the absence of changes in glucocorticoid levels (Jessop et al. 1987; Moynihan et al. 1989). Further, elevated corticosteroid levels are not always associated with altered immune function (Mormede et al. 1988; Flores et al. 1990).

Opioids have been implicated in the modulation of host defense responses in a wide range of species (Faisal et al. 1989; Stefano et al. 1990; Shavit 1991). As with glucocorticoids, investigations of the role of opioids in stress-induced immune alterations show that the relationship is complex. Opioid-mediated analgesia can result in decreased NK cell cytotoxic responses (Shavit et al. 1984; Cunnick et al. 1988; Keller et al. 1988; Rabin et al. 1990), and decreased survival following tumor challenge (Lewis et al. 1983). However, high levels of β-endorphins do not always result in decreased NK cell function (Flores et al. 1990), and stress-induced changes in NK cell activity may occur in the absence of opioid involvement (Ben-Eliyahu et al. 1990).

As to the participation of neuropeptides in various responses to stress, hypothalamic neurons producing corticotropin-releasing hormone and neuronal as well as adenohypophysial cells furnishing peptides derived from proopiomelanocortin i.e., adrenocorticortropic hormone, melanocyte-stimulating hormone, and endorphin can be listed. In addition, various neuropeptides, including enkephalins, are released by cells of the immune system.

Experimentally induced stress provides information on additional regulatory substances with which neuropeptides must interact. The sympathetic nervous system is activated by stressor administration, and there is good evidence that catecholamines are immunoregulatory (Madden and Livnat 1991). Increased epinephrine following physical exertion in humans is correlated with decreased $CD4/CD8^+$ T-cell and decreased T/B-cell ratios (Landmann et al. 1984). Further, chemical sympathectomy with 6-hydroxydopamine prior to restraint stress in mice prevents some but not all stress-induced immune alterations (Okimura et al. 1986c).

Changes in gamma-aminobutyric acid receptor binding in the brain occur following stressor administration (Biggio et al. 1981), and benzodiazepine "inverse agonists" that mimic stress responses can result in suppression of NK cell activity (Petitto et al. 1989). Okimura and Nigo (1986) reported that administration of the anti-anxiolytic compound diazapam prior to restraint of mice prevents the stress-induced suppression of antibody responses. However, Cunnick et al. (1988) reported that diazepam has no effect on footshock-induced suppression of splenic mitogen or NK cell responses.

In summary, the data collected from studies linking stressors to neuroendocrine changes and resulting immune alteration suggest that different neuroendocrine and additional mechanisms may affect different immune responses following administration of different stressors. The observed changes in an immune response following stressor application are certainly due to interactions among a number of neurohormones and transmitters that undoubtedly have associated diurnal rhythms. Therefore, all attempts to determine the mechanisms of stress-induced alterations of immune responses must also take into account the circadian rhythms associated with the signal molecules that modulate immune function (Richardson and Martin 1988). A complete understanding of the mechanisms resulting in stress-induced immune modulation may well remain elusive for some time since, as has been discussed, there are reasons to believe that different stressors have different effects on different parameters of immunity, and that multiple pathways can be invoked to elicit adaptive responses on the part of the organism.

Acknowledgements. The work of the authors cited in this manuscript was funded by NIMH 45681. RA is funded by MH 06318.

References

Ader R, Cohen N (1985) CNS-immune system interactions: conditioning phenomena. Behav Brain Sci 8:379–394

Ader R, Cohen N (1991) The influence of conditioning on immune responses. In Ader R, Cohen N, Felten DL (eds) Psychoneuroimmunology. 2nd edn. Academic Press, New York, pp 611–646

Ader R, Friedman SB (1965) Differential early experiences and the susceptibility to transplanted tumors. J Comp Physiol Psych 59:361–374

Ader R, Felten DL, Cohen N (1990) Interactions between the brain and the immune system. Annu Rev Pharmacol Toxicol 30:561–602

Beden SN, Brain PF (1982) Studies on the effect of social stress on measures of disease resistance in laboratory mice. Aggress Behav 8:126–129

Beden SN, Brain PF (1984) Effects of attack-related stress on the primary immune response to sheep red blood cells in castrated mice. IRCS Med Sci 12:675

Ben-Eliyahu S, Yirmiya R, Shavit Y, Liebeskind JC (1990) Stress-induced suppression of natural killer cell cytotoxicity in the rat: a naltrexone-insensitive paradigm. Behav Neurosci 104:235–238

Bernton EW, Bryant HU, Holaday JW (1991) Prolactin and immune function. In: Ader R, Cohen N, Felten DL (eds) Psychoneuroimmunology, 2nd edn, Academic Press, New York, pp 403–428

Biggio G, Corda MG, Demontis G, Rossetti Z, Gessa GL (1981) Rapid changes in GABA binding induced by stress in different areas of the brain. Brain Res. 229:363–369

Blalock JE (1988) Production of neuroendocrine peptide hormones by the immune system. In: Blalock JE, Bost KL (eds) Neuroimmunoendocrin. Karger, New York, pp 1–13 (Progress in allergy, vol 43)

Blecha F, Barry RA, Kelley KW (1982a) Stress-induced alterations in delayed-type hypersensitivity to SRBC and contact sensitivity to DNFB in mice. Proc Soc Exp Biol Med 169:239–246

Blecha F, Kelley KW, Satteriee DG (1982b) Adrenal involvement in the expression of delayed-type hypersensitivity to SRBC and contact sensitivity to DNFB in stressed mice. Proc Soc Exp Biol Med 169:247–252

Bly JE, Miller NW, Clem LW (1990) A monoclonal antibody specific for neutrophils in normal and stressed channel catfish. Dev Comp Immunol 14:211–221

Brenner GJ, Cohen N, Ader R, Moynihan JA (1990) Increased pulmonary metastases in mice following handling. Life Sci 47:1813–1819

Carr DJJ, Blalock JE (1991) Neuropeptide hormones and receptors common to the immune and neuroendocrine systems: bidirectional pathways of intersystem communication. In: Ader R, Cohen N, Felten D L (eds) Psychoneuroimmunology, 2nd edn Academic Press, New York, pp 573–588

Coe CL, Rosenberg LT, Fisher M, Levine S (1987) Psychological factors capable of preventing the inhibition of antibody responses in separated infant monkeys. Child Dev 58:1420–1430

Coffey RG, Hadden JW (1985) Neurotransmitters, hormones, and cyclic nucleotides in lymphocyte regulation. Fed Proc 44:112–117

Cohen S, Williamson GM (1991) Stress and infectious disease in humans. Psych Bull 109:5–24

Cunnick JE, Lysle DT, Armfield A, Rabin BS (1988) Shock-induced modulation of lymphocyte responsiveness and natural killer activity: differential mechanisms of induction. Brain Behav Immun 2:102–113

Dantzer R, Kelley KW (1989) Stress and immunity: an integrated view of relationships between the brain and the immune system. Life Sci 44:1995–2008

Edwards EA, Rahe RH, Stephens PM, Henry JP (1980) Antibody response to bovine serum albumin in mice: the effects of psychosocial environmental change. Proc Soc Exp Biol Med 164:478–481

Ellsaesser CF, Clem LW (1986) Haematological and immunological changes in channel catfish stressed by handling and transport. J Fish Biol 28:511–521

Ellsaesser CF, Clem LW (1987) Cortisol-induced hematologic and immunologic changes in channel catfish (*Ictalurus punctatus*) Comp Biochem Physiol 87A:405–408

Esterling B, Rabin BS (1987) Stress-induced alteration of T-lymphocyte subsets and humoral immunity in mice. Behav Neurosci 101:115–119

Faisal M, Chiapelli F, Ahmed II, Cooper EL, Weiner H (1989) Social confrontation "stress" in aggressive fish is associated with an endogenous opioid-mediated suppression of proliferative responses, to mitogens and nonspecific cytotoxicity. Brain Behav Immune 3:223–233

Feldbush TL, Stunz LL, Lafrenz DE (1986) Memory B-cell activation, differentiation, and isotype switching. In: Cambier JC (ed) B-Lymphocyte differentiation, CRC Press, Boca Raton, pp 135–162

Felten SY, Felten DL (1991) The innervation of lymphoid tissue. In: Ader R, Cohen N, Felten DL (eds) Psychoneuroimmunology, 2nd edn. Academic Press, New York, pp 27–70

Fleshner M, Laudenslager ML, Simons L, Maier SF (1989) Reduced serum antibodies associated with social defeat in rats. Physiol Behav 45:1183–1187

Flores CM, Hernandez MC, Hargreaves KM, Bayer BM (1990) Restraint stress-induced elevations in plasma corticosterone and beta-endorphin are not accompanied by alterations in immune function. J Neuroimmunol 28:219–225

Ghoneum M, Gill G, Assanah P, Stevens W (1987) Susceptibility of natural killer cell activity of old rats to stress. Immunology 60:461–465

Ghoneum M, Faisal M, Peters G, Ahmed II, Cooper EL (1988) Suppression of natural cytotoxic cell activity by social aggressiveness in *Tilapia*. Dev Comp Immunol 12:595–602

Glaser R, Rice J, Sheridan J, Fertel R, Stout J, Speicher C, Pinsky D, Kotur M, Post A, Beck M, Kiecolt-Glaser J (1987) Stress-related immune suppression: health implications. Brain Behav Immun 1:7–20

Gorsczynski R (1991) Conditioned immunosuppression: analysis of lymphocytes and host environment of young and aged mice. In: Ader R, Cohen N, Felten DL (eds) Psychoneuroimmunology, 2nd edn. Academic Press, New York, pp 647–662

Hall NRS, O'Grady MP, Farah JM (1991) Thymic hormones and immune function: Mediation via neuroendocrine circuits. In: Ader R, Cohen N, Felten DL (eds) Psychoneuroimmunology, 2nd edn. Academic Press, New York, pp 515–528

Hardy C, Quay J, Livnat S, Ader R (1990) Altered T-lymphocyte response following aggressive encounters in mice. Physiol Behav 47:1245–1251

Heijen CJ, Kavelaars A, Ballieux RE (1991) Corticotropin-releasing hormone and proopiomelanocortin-derived peptides in the modulation of immune function. In: Ader R, Cohen N, Felten DL (eds) Psychoneuroimmunology, 2nd edn. Academic Press, New York, pp 429–446

Ito Y, Mine K, Ago Y, Nakagawa T, Fujiwara M, Ueki E (1983) Attack stress and IgE antibody response in rats. Pharmacol Biochem Behav 19:883–886

Jessop JJ, Gale K, Bayer BM (1987) Enhancement of rat lymphocyte proliferation after prolonged exposure to stress. J Neuroimmunol 16:261–271

Johnson HM, Torres BA (1985) Regulation of lymphokine production by arginine vasopressin and oxytocin: modulation of lymphocyte function by neurohypophyseal hormones. J Immunol 135:773s–778s

Khansari DN, Murgo AJ, Faith RE (1990) Effects of stress on the immune system. Immunol Today 11:170–175

Keller SE, Weiss JM, Schleifer SJ, Miller NE, Stein M (1981) Suppression of immunity by stress: effects of a graded series of stressors on lymphocyte stimulation in rat. Science 213:1397–1400

Keller SE, Weiss JM, Schleifer SJ, Miller NE, Stein M (1983) Stress-induced suppression of immunity in adrenalectomized rats. Science 221:1301–1304

Keller SE, Schleifer SJ, Stein M (1984) Stress-induced suppression of lymphocyte function in rats. In: Cooper EL (ed) Stress immunity, and aging. Dekker, New York, pp 109–121

Keller SE, Schleifer SJ, Liotta AS, Bond RN, Farhoody N, Stein M (1988) Stress-induced alterations of immunity in hypophysectomized rats. Proc Natl Acad Sci USA 85:9297–9301

Kelley KW (1991) Growth hormone in immunobiology. In: Ader R, Cohen N, Felten DL (eds) Psychoneuroimmunology, 2nd edn. Academic Press, New York, pp 377–402

Kemeny ME, Solomon GF, Morley JE, Bennett TL (1994) Psychoneuroimmunology. In: Nemeroff CB (ed) A comprehensive textbook of neuroendocrinology

Khansari DN, Murgo AJ, Faith RE (1990) Effects of stress on the immune system. Immunol Today 11:170–175

Landmann RMA, Muller FB, Perini C, Wesp M, Erne P, Buhler FR (1984) Changes of immunoregulatory cells induced by psychological and physical stress: relationship to plasma catecholamines. Clin Exp Immunol 58:127–135

Laudenslager ML, Ryan SM, Drugan RC, Hyson RL, Maier SF (1983) Coping and immunosuppression: inescapable but not escapable shock suppresses lymphocyte proliferation. Science 221:568–570

Laudenslager M, Fleshner M, Hofstadter P, Held PE, Simons L, Maier F (1988) Suppression of specific antibody production by inescapable shock: stability under varying conditions. Brain Behav Immun 2:92–101

Lewis JW, Shavit Y, Terman GW, Gale RP, Liebeskind JC (1983) Stress and morphine affect survival of rats challenged with a mammary ascites tumor (MAT 1 3762IS). Nat Immun Cell Growth Regul 3:43–50

Lown BA, Dutka ME (1987) Early handling enhances mitogen responses of splenic cells in adult C3H mice. Brain Behav Immun 1:356–360

Lysle DT, Lyte M, Fowler H, Rabin BS (1987) Shock-induced modulation of lymphocyte reactivity: suppression, habituation, and recovery. Life Sci 41:1805–1814

Lysle DT, Cunnick JE, Fowier H, Rani ISS (1988) Pavlovian conditioning of shock-induced suppression of lymphocyte reactivity: acquisition, extinction, and preexposure effects. Life Sci 42:2185–2194

Madden KS, Livnat S (1991) Catecholamine action and immunologic reactivity In: Ader R, Cohen N, Felten DL (eds) Psychoneuroimmunology, 2nd edn. Academic Press, New York, pp 283–310

Maestroni GJM, Conti A (1991) Role of the pineal neurohormone melatonin in the psychoneuroendocrine-immune network. In: Ader R, Cohen N, Felten DL (eds) Psychoneuroimmunology, 2nd edn. Academic Press, New York, pp 495–514

Maier SF, Laudenslager ML (1988) Inescapable shock, shock controllability, and mitogen-stimulated lymphocyte proliferation. Brain Behav Immun 2:87–91

McCruden AB, Stimson WH (1991) Sex hormones and immune function. In: Ader R, Cohen N, Felten DL (eds) Psychoneuroimmunology, 2nd edn. Academic Press, New York, pp 474–494

McGillis JP, Mitsuhashi M, Payan DG (1991) Immunologic properties of substance P. In: Ader R, Cohen N, Felten DL (eds) Psychoneuroimmunology, 2nd edn. Academic Press, New York, pp 209–224

Michaut R, Dechambre R, Doumerc S, Lesourd IS, Devillechabrolle A, Moulias R (1980) Influence of early maternal deprivation on adult humoral immune response in mice. Physiol Behav 26:189–191

Monjan AA, Collector MI (1977) Stress-induced modulation of the immune response. Science 196:307–308

Mormede P, Dantzer R, Michaud B, Kelley K, Le Moal M (1988) Influence of stressor predictability and behavioral control on lymphocyte reactivity, antibody responses, and neuroendocrine activation in rats. Physiol Behav 43:577–583

Moynihan JA, Cohen N (1992) Stress and immunity. In: Schneiderman N, Baum A (eds) Stress and disease processes: prospectives in behavioral medicine. Lawrence Erlbaum, Hillsdale, N J, pp 27–48

Moynihan JA, Koota D, Brenner G, Cohen N, Ader R (1989) Repeated intraperitoneal injections of saline attenuate the antibody response to a subsequent intraperitoneal injection of antigen. Brain Behav Immun 3:90–96

Moynihan J, Brenner G, Koota D, Breneman S, Cohen N, Ader R (1990a) The effects of handling on antibody production, mitogen responses, spleen cell number, and lymphocyte subpopulations. Life Sci 46:1937–1944

Moynihan JA, Ader R, Grota LJ, Schachtman TR, Cohen N (1990b) The effects of stress on the development of immunological memory following low-dose antigen priming in mice. Brain Behav Immun 4:1–12

Moynihan JA, Brenner GJ, Ader R, Cohen N (1991) The effects of handling on immunologic processes. Ann NY Acad Sci 650:262–267

Munck A, Guyre PM (1991) Glucocorticoids and immune function. In: Ader R, Cohen N, Felten DL (eds) Psychoneuroimmunology, 2nd edn. Academic Press, New York, 447–474

Newton G, Bly CG, McCrary M (1962) Effects of early experience on the response to transplantable tumor. J Nerv Mental Dis 134:522–527

Okimura T, Nigo Y (1986) Stress and immune responses. I Suppression of T-cell functions in restraint-stressed mice. Jpn J Phamacol 40:505–511

Okimura T, Satomi-Sasaki, Ohkuma S (1986a) Stress and immune responses. II Identification of stress-sensitive cells in murine spleen cells. Jpn J Pharmacol 40:513–525

Okimura T, Ogawa M, Yamauchi T (1986b) Stress and immune responses, III. Effect of restraint stress on delayed type hypersensitivity (DTH) response, natural killer (NK) activity, and phagocytosis in mice. Jpn J Pharmacol 41:229–235

Okimura T, Ogawa M, Yamauchi T, Sasaki Y (1986c) Stress and immune responses IV. Adrenal involvement in the alteration of antibody responses in restraint-stressed mice. Jpn J Pharmacol 41:237–245

Ottaway CA (1991) Vasoactive intestinal peptide and immune function. In: Ader R, Cohen N, Felten DL (eds) Psychoneuroimmunology, 2nd edn. Academic Press, New York, pp 225–262

Peters G, Schwarzer R (1985) Changes in hematopoietic tissue of rainbow trout under influence of stress. Dis Aquat Orig 1:1–10

Petitto JM, Skolnick P, Arora PK (1989) Suppression of natural killer cell activity by FG 7142, a benzodiazepine receptor "inverse agonist." Brain Behav Immunol 3:39–46

Rabin BS, Salvin SB (1987) Effect of differential housing and time on immune reactivity to sheep erythrocytes and Candida. Brain Behav Immun 1:267–275

Rabin BS, Lyte M, Epstein LH, Caggiula AR (1987) Alteration of immune competency by number of mice housed per cage. Ann NY Acad Sci 496:492–500

Rabin BS, Cohen S, Ganguli R, Lysle DT, Cunnick JE (1989) Bidirectional interaction between the central nervous system and the immune system. Crit Rev Immunol 9:279–312

Rabin BS, Cunnick JE, Lysle DT (1990) Stress-induced alteration of immune function. Prog Neuroendocrinimmunol 3:116–124

Raymond LN, Reyes E, Tokuda S, Jones BC (1986) Differential immune response in two handled inbred strains of mice. Physiol Behav 37:295–297

Richardson GS, Martin JB (1988) Circadian rhythyms in neuroendocrinolgy and immunology: influence of aging. Prog Neuroendocrinimmunol 1:16–20

Selye H (1950) General physiology and pathology of systemic stress. In: Stress. ACTA, Montreal, p 5–51

Shavit Y (1991) Stress-induced immune modulation in animals: opiates and endogenous opioid peptides. In: Ader R, Cohen N, Felten DL (eds) Psychoneuroimmunology, 2nd edn, Academic Press, New York, pp 789–805

Shavit Y, Lewis JW, Terman GW, Gale RP, Liebeskind JC (1984) Opioid peptides mediate the suppressive effect of stress on natural killer cell cytotoxicity. Science 223:188–190

Shavit Y, Terman GW, Lewis JW, Zane CJ, Gale RP, Liebeskind JC (1986) Effects of footshock stress and morphine on natural killer lymphocytes in rats: studies of tolerance and cross-tolerance. Brain Res 372:382–385

Sklar LS, Anisman H (1981) Stress and cancer. Psych Bull 89:369–406

Solomon GF (1969) Stress and antibody response in rats. Int Arch Allergy 35:97–104

Solomon GF, Levine S, Kraft JK (1968) Early experience and immunity. Nature 220:821–822

Stanisz AM, Befus D, Bienenstock J (1986) Differential effects of vasoactive intestinal peptide, substance P and somatostatin on immunoglobulin synthesis, and proliferation by lymphocytes from Peyer's patches, mesenteric lymph nodes, and spleen. J Immunol 136:152–156

Stefano G B, Cadet P, Dokun A, Scharrer B (1990) A neuroimmunoregulatory-like mechanism responding to stress in the marine bivalve Mytilus edulis. Brain Behav Immun 4:1–6

Steplewski Z, Vogel WH (1986) Total leukocytes, T cell subpopulation, and natural killer (NK) cell activity in rats exposed to restraint stress. Life Sci 38:2419–2427

Steplewski Z, Vogel WH, Ehya H, Poropatich C, Smith JM (1985) Effects of restraint stress on inoculated tumor growth and immune response in rats. Cancer Res 45:5126–5133

Tripp RA, Maule AG, Schreck CB, Kaattari SL (1987) Cortisol mediated suppression of salmonid lymphocyte responses in vitro. Dev Comp Immunol 11:565–576

Vessey SH (1964) Effects of grouping on levels of circulating antibodies in mice. Proc Soc Exp Biol Med 115:252–255

Wedemeyer G (1970) The role of stress in the disease resistance of fishes. In: Snieszko SF (ed) A symposium on diseases of fish and shellfishes, special Publication, vol 5. American Fisheries Society, Washington DC, pp 30–35

Zalcman S, Minkiewicz-Janda A, Richter M, Anisman H (1988) Critical periods associated with stressor effects on antibody titers and on the plaque-forming cell response to sheep red blood cells. Brain Behav Immun 2:254–266

Zalcman S, Richter M, Anisman H (1989) Alterations of immune functioning following exposure to stressor related cues. Brain Behav Immun 3:99–110

Pharmacological and Binding Evidence for Opioid Receptors on Vertebrate and Invertebrate Blood Cells

G. B. Stefano

Introduction

Current evidence indicates that opioid peptides, whose roles in the nervous system are well established, affect immunoactive cells (Smith and Blalock 1981; for review see Blalock 1989). The significance of this phenomenon is highlighted by the discovery that it applies to invertebrates as well as vertebrates (Leung and Stefano 1987; Stefano 1982, 1989). A search for stereoselective mechanisms mediating these neuropeptide activities has been under way for some time. Its results, though still incomplete, seem to indicate that in both groups of animals the complexity of ligand-receptor binding is greater than anticipated. The existing evidence for these parallels presented in this chapter, and in that by Janković and Marić, is based on pharmacological data as well as binding studies.

Pharmacological Evidence for the Presence of Opioid Receptors

Vertebrates

In recent years much information has been obtained on the pharmacological effects of opiate and opioid substances on mammalian immunocompetent cells. Since the first studies of Wybran et al. (1979) reporting that Met-enkephalin heightens the formation of active T-cell rosettes there have been many additional reports. Similar effects were seen with Leu-enkephalin. The percent of T-lymphocytes forming active rosettes was increased by β-endorphin in normal human donors and lymphoma patients (Miller et al. 1983). McCain et al. (1982) demonstrated that in vitro β-endorphin (10^{-7} M) suppresses the blastogenic response of human blood lymphocytes to phytohemagglutinin (PHA), and that this effect is not blocked by 10^{-6} M naloxone. Treatment with naloxone alone had no effect on PHA mitogenesis. According to Gilman et al. (1982), lymphocyte proliferation is enhanced by β-endorphin in rat spleen lymphocytes with only a

Multidisciplinary Center for the Study of Aging, Old Westbury Neuroscience Research Institute, State University of New York, College at Old Westbury, Old Westbury, NY 11568–0210, USA

Scharrer et al. (Eds.)
Neuropeptides and Immunoregulation

slight suppressive effect by naloxone, and β-endorphin has no effect on the B-cell mitogen, lipopolysaccharide/dextran sulfate. Leu- and Met-enkephalin also enhance lymphocyte proliferation in mouse spleen lymphocytes (Plotnikoff and Miller 1983).

β-Endorphin, Met-enkephalin, and γ-endorphin enhance cellular cytotoxicity in human natural killer (NK) cells against the NK-sensitive K562 cell line, and naloxone blocks this effect (Mathews et al. 1983; Faith et al. 1984; Kay et al. 1984). Yamasaki et al. (1983) demonstrated that various opioid substances (β-endorphin, Met-enkephalin) can prevent the prostaglandin E_1 (PGE_1) mediated release from rat mast cells. At the same time, opioids have been shown to enhance flare reactions in the skin as well as to increase the itch associated with histamine release (Fjellner and Hagermark 1982; Casale et al. 1984).

Enkephalin administration to male Wistar rats decreased the level of IgE, and caused degranulation of mast cells and precipitation of anti-ovalbumin antibodies (Marić and Janković 1988). These results strongly suggest that enkephalins act to suppress antibody production and to sensitize mast cells with specific IgE, thus exerting an antianaphylactic reaction. In another study it was shown that both Met- and Leu-enkephalin enhance a plaque-forming cell response and hemagglutinin production. The end result of the study indicated that this response is mediated via δ- and μ-opioid receptors. This conclusion was based on differential sensitivities to naloxone and a moderately potent δ ligand, ICI 174864 (Janković and Marić 1988). However, in order to achieve a clear opioid receptor-type classification more ligands should have been tested (see also Janković and Marić, this volume).

Pretreatment of peritoneal macrophages of rats with Met-enkephalin enhances, in a naloxone-reversible manner, the lysis of antibody target cells (Foris et al. 1984). It is of interest to note that there is also enhanced superoxide synthesis; however, naloxone blockade of this effect was not reported. In another contribution, Sharp et al. (1985) demonstrated enhanced superoxide production in both macrophages (1 μM) and polymorphonuclear leukocytes (1–100 pM) with dynorphin and β-endorphin, an effect antagonized by naloxone. Unfortunately, the experiments did not include a treatment with naloxone alone, since others have shown that naloxone may have mixed agonist–antagonist properties (Brown et al. 1986; Stefano et al. 1989a).

β-Endorphin and various opiates were found to enhance calcium binding in rat peritoneal mast cells in a naloxone sensitive manner (Liu et al. 1983). Opioids also have been implicated in mast-cell degranulation and the data tentatively suggest the presence of κ- and ε-opioid receptor subtypes (Casale et al. 1984).

Opioid treatment of mouse splenocytes decreases the number of cells producing antibodies (Johnson et al. 1982; Heijnen et al. 1986). Naloxone blockage of this activity has been demonstrated (Johnson et al. 1982). It is of special interest that β-endorphin has been shown to be ineffective, suggesting that δ-type opioid receptors mediate this pharmacological effect. β-Endorphin has been reported to increase the incorporation of thymidine into PHA-stimulated interleukin-2 (IL-2) dependent human T-lymphocytes and to reverse the proliferative responses initiated by PGE_2 (Farrar 1984).

T-cell rosetting is inhibited by morphine in a naloxone-reversible manner (De Carolis et al. 1984). Mononuclear cell cytotoxicity in peripheral blood is enhanced by opioids in a naloxone-reversible manner (Mathews et al. 1983; Froelich and Bankhurst 1984; Kay et al. 1984). The effect is accompanied by enhanced recruitment of stem NK effector cells. Subsequently, the active material believed to cause this effect was shown to be in the supernatant and blockable by naloxone (Wybran 1985; Mandler et al. 1986). In another interesting study, Shavit et al. (1984, 1986) demonstrated that the NK activity of splenocytes taken from rats given footshock is decreased. They found that the type of analgesia produced by different footshock procedures is correlated with the decrease in NK cell cytotoxicity. Additionally, they demonstrated an associated increase in the growth of implanted tumors (Shavit et al. 1985). Stefano et al. (1989a, b) demonstrated that D-Ala^2-Met^5-enkephalin (DAMA) is the most potent opioid ligand inducing morphometric changes indicative of cellular activation in human granulocytes (Table 1). The important role of Met-enkephalin suggested by these results is further supported by the information presented by Scharrer and Stefano and by Janković and Marić (both in this volume). In summary, there is strong pharmacological evidence for the presence of opioid receptors, and of various opioid receptor subtypes on specific mammalian immunoresponsive cells.

Table 1. Displacement of [^{3}H]DAMA (1 n*M*) by opioid ligands in human and *Mytilus* immunocyte membrane suspensions (from Stefano et al. 1992a)

Ligand		IC_{50} n*M*	
		Human granulocytes	*Mytilus* immunocytes
δ			
	DAMA	0.6	0.6
	Deltorphin	0.5	0.5
	*Met-enkephalin	0.7	0.9
	DADLE	6.2	7.7
	DPDPE	8.1	10.4
μ			
	DAGO	12.3	16.5
κ			
	dynorphin 1–17	21.2	19.3
Antagonists			
	Naloxone	15.6	22.7
	Naltrexone	1.1	1.0

*Incubations with Met-enkephalin contained phosphoramidon (100 m*M*) and bestatin (100 μ*M*) to inhibit enzyme action (7, 9, 17). For other details, see text. DADLE, (D-Ala^2, Leu^5)-enkephalin; DPDPE, (D-Pen^2, D-Pen^5)-enkephalin; DAGO, (D-Ala^2, $MePhe^4$, $Gly(ol)^5$)-enkephalin.

Invertebrates

Evidence for the presence of opioid receptors on the immunocompetent cells of the mollusc *Mytilus edulis* and the insect *Leucophaea maderae* has been obtained by determining the effects of exogenous opioids on various cellular activities in the presence or absence of naloxone (Stefano et al. 1989b; Scharrer and Stefano, this volume). In vitro and in vivo experiments have demonstrated that adherence and directed migratory activity of immunoresponsive hemocytes are enhanced in the presence of the stable methionine enkephalin analog DAMA (Stefano et al. 1989a). Opioid-activated immunocytes exhibit the same conformational changes (flattening, development of pseudopodia, etc.) as those of their mammalian counterparts (Falke and Fisher 1986). A comparison of the stimulatory effects of DAMA with those observed in the presence of related neuropeptides and non-peptide substances (Table 1) reveals that also in the invertebrates tested DAMA is the most potent substance examined thus far. Moreover, a grouping of the results according to binding preference shows that eight ligands tested in *Mytilus* are molecules that respond more or less selectively to specific types of receptors.

Whereas heterogeneity of receptor subtypes in the mammalian immune system is fairly well established (see Stefano 1989), no corresponding information on this problem in invertebrates had been available until very recently. Most of the substances tested (Table 1), including δ-, μ-, and κ-selective ligands, elicited responses at concentrations no lower than 10^{-9} *M*. DAMA was the only ligand that was most effective at a concentration as low as 10^{-11} *M* without a specific enzyme inhibitor present to prevent proteolytic attack (Shipp et al. 1990). It is of particular significance that DAMA proved to be equally potent in the tests with *Mytilus* blood cells as in those with human leukocytes (Stefano et al. 1989b). The distinctly lower effectiveness of the closely related δ-opioid ligand DADLE in both human and invertebrate immune reactions is in contrast to the "classical" situation in the mammalian nervous system, where this discrepancy in binding potency does not exist. An observation supporting the distinctive role of Met-enkephalin in immunoregulation is the high potency of this opioid in granulocyte-endothelial cell interactions demonstrated in human umbilical veins (Boogaerts et al. 1983). The high degree of specificity of DAMA suggests a distinctive role for Met-enkephalin in immunoregulatory processes and the possible existence of a special subtype of δ-receptor responsive to this ligand (Stefano et al. 1989b). This possibility has subsequently been substantiated (see below).

In vitro tests with Met-enkephalin revealed the same high-potency values as those obtained with DAMA, but only in the presence of an enzyme inhibitor (phosphoramidon), since this pentapeptide is downregulated by neutral endopeptidase 24.11 in both human and *Mytilus* immunoresponsive cells (Shipp et al. 1990; Scharrer and Stefano, this volume).

Stereospecific Opioid Receptor Binding

Mammalian Cells

There have been several reports characterizing stereospecific binding of opioid peptides to respective receptors on various mammalian blood cells. Opiate/opioid receptors are believed to occur on phagocytic leukocytes (Lopker et al. 1980), lymphocytes and platelets (Mehrishi and Mills 1983), human T-lymphocytes (Ausciello and Roda 1984), and polymorphonuclear leukocytes (Falke and Fischer 1985). Furthermore, opioid peptides may modulate lymphokine activity in vertebrates (Farrar 1984) and invertebrates (Stefano et al. 1992b).

A crucial criterion for the demonstration of opioid binding, namely stereospecificity, was accounted for in only two of these studies (Lopker et al. 1980; Falke and Fischer 1985). Moreover, in the Lopker et al. (1980) study certain data relevant to the issue were not presented, and in the Falke and Fischer (1985) study the difference observed between the active and inactive naloxone enantiomers was much smaller than normally expected in such an analysis. The results of the Farrar (1984) study were quite complex in view of the small number of ligands tested. The author attributed the complexity to the possible existence of multiple opioid receptor subtypes; yet the results did not reveal a familiar pattern. It is of interest to note that in a few of the available reports dissociation constants were said to have been calculated as well as the number of binding sites per cell (Lopker et al. 1980; Johnson et al. 1982); however, the results of these calculations were not presented. In another binding study the internalization of β-endorphin was proposed (Falke and Fischer 1986). However, missing information, namely the lack of a binding isotherm or a typical competition curve, questions the significance of the phenomenon.

Carr et al. (1988a) reported the presence of δ-opioid receptors on human and murine leukocytes based on the specific effect of *cis*-(+)-3-methylfentanylisothiocyanate (Superfit) as well as naloxone sensitivity. The authors tested various δ- and μ-type ligands in their analysis of binding by polyacrylamide gel electrophoresis coupled to autoradiography. They presented hard evidence to suggest that gross binding and its sensitivity to various ligands occur. The occurrence of opioid binding sites on murine splenocyte membranes was also investigated (Carr et al. 1988b). The experiment was performed by cross-linking ^{125}I-labeled β-endorphin to splenocyte membranes, with and without naloxone in the medium, by subjecting the membrane extracts to sodium dodecyl sulfate polyacrylamide gel electrophoresis and to autoradiography. It is noteworthy to mention that these authors also demonstrated that β-endorphin binding reduces potassium conductance, possibly by reducing the size of the channel openings for this ion. Thus, this significant study demonstrated stereospecific binding which apparently is associated with a specific ionophoric domain.

More recently, Radulescu et al. (1991) demonstrated a μ-class of opioid binding site on lymphocytes. This binding site under nonreducing conditions has a molecular weight of 58 kDa and under reducing conditions one of 70 kDa. The binding site is also coupled to calcium uptake pathways. Thus, lymphocytes possess a specific binding site resembling that of the opioid μ-subtype.

In a review of opioid binding to various immunocompetent cells, Sibinga and Goldstein (1988) came to a conclusion shared by the author (Stefano 1989) in regard to the tentative nature of some of these opioid-binding reports. This evaluation is based on knowledge of the detailed requirements for defining a high-affinity binding site, and for declaring it to be a stereospecific receptor only if the binding can be correlated with a specific function. In general, many of the earlier studies referred to suffer from a lack of selecting proper ligands, obeying the "protocol" for a standard binding assay, demonstrating saturability and stereospecificity, and an in depth understanding of how much information the apparent affinities can yield for the elucidation of possible subtypes of opioid receptors. Important omissions in some of the reports summarized here lead to the conclusion that present data are largely preliminary but nevertheless very promising.

A recent study (Stefano et al. 1992a) examined the effects of the opioid neuropeptide (D-Ala^2) deltorphin I, isolated from amphibian skin, on various immunoregulatory activities. This endogenous amphibian heptapeptide – Tyr-[D-Ala^2]-Phe-Asp-Val-Val-Gly-NH_2; (D-Ala^2) deltorphin I – which according to Erspamer et al. (1990) has a high potency, revealed a high affinity and selectivity for δ-opioid binding sites on human granulocytes and invertebrate immunocytes. Like DAMA, it stimulated the activity of these immune cells at a concentration of 10^{-11} M in a naloxone-sensitive manner.

The opioid receptor presumed to be involved in this activity was biochemically characterized as follows. In cold saturation experiments a single high-affinity binding site was revealed with a K_d of 0.45 nM and a B_{max} of 3.78 pmol/g membrane protein for human granulocytes (Fig. 1). Hill analysis revealed a coefficient of 0.976. Pretreatment of granulocyte membranes with increasing concentrations of DALCE (a select δ-opioid antagonist), like that of rat membranes (Bowen et al. 1987), significantly blocked [^{3}H]DPDPE binding to δ-opioid sites. By contrast, the same treatment of granulocyte membranes with DALCE did not significantly affect the binding of [^{3}H](D-Ala^2) deltorphin I or [^{3}H]DAMA. Therefore, a special receptor (δ_2) can be postulated to mediate these two opioid activities.

Invertebrates

Since DAMA is potent in initiating immunocyte conformational alterations, as noted above and by Scharrer and Stefano (this volume), it is the ligand of preference in the search for opioid binding sites. In *Mytilus* immunocyte membrane suspensions a single high-affinity [^{3}H]DAMA binding profile became evident upon Scatchard analysis (Fig. 2). This high-affinity site exhibited a K_d of 0.8 nM with a B_{max} of 4 pmol/mg protein. Interestingly, in repetitive assays using glass-on-glass homogenization the K_d remained relatively constant whereas the

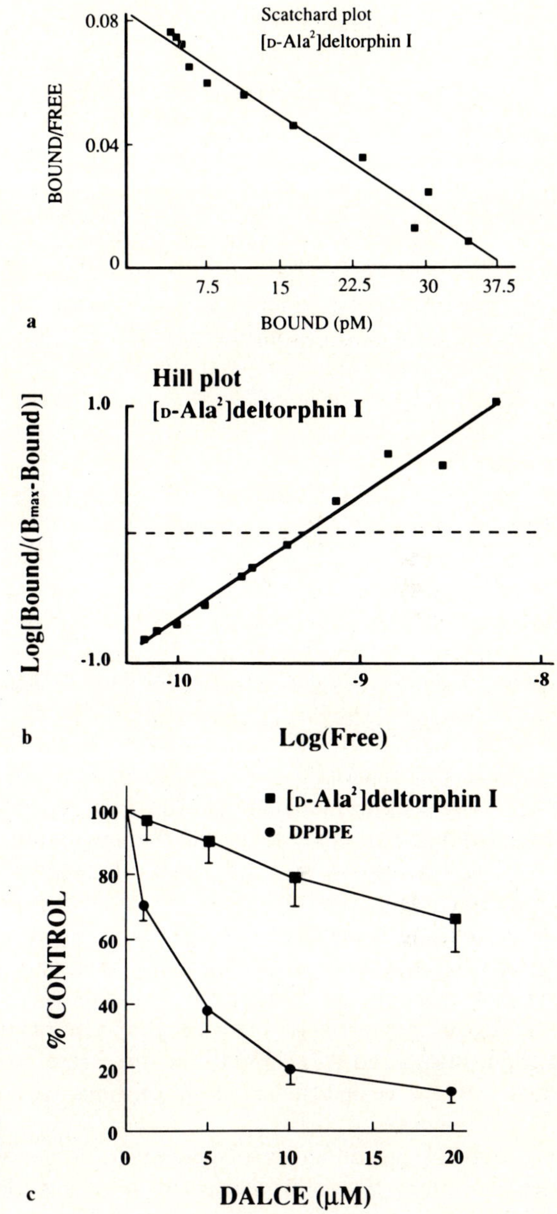

Fig. 1a–c. Binding of [^{3}H]deltorphin to human granulocytes. **a** Scatchard analysis. **b** Hill analysis. **c** Displacement

B_{max} appeared to vary (0.9–8.0). This same observation was made in tests with human granulocytes (B_{max} 2.0–8.0). Furthermore, if a polytron was used to homogenize the various cells, it was frequently impossible to find specific binding. This may all serve to demonstrate that immunocyte opioid receptors may be extremely sensitive to physical disturbances. It may also explain the inability of

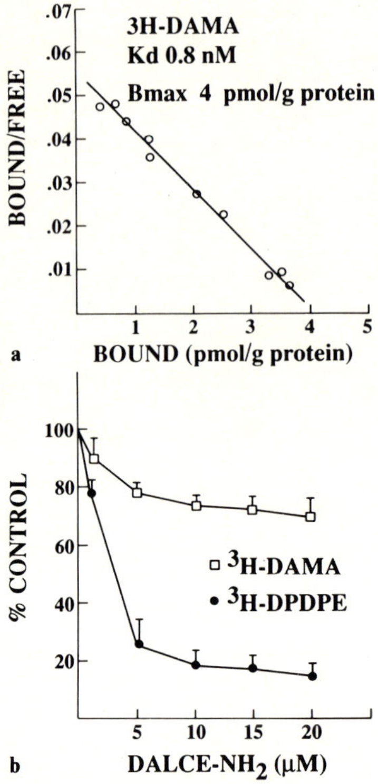

Fig. 2a, b. Binding analysis of [^{3}H]DAMA to *Mytilus* immunocyte membrane suspensions. **a** Scatchard analysis. **b** Displacement analysis

various investigators to demonstrate highly specific stereospecific opioid binding sites (Sibinga and Goldstein 1988; Stefano 1989).

The preincubation of *Mytilus* immunocyte membranes with DALCE, as compared with those in human granulocytes, had the following results. There was a marked concentration-dependent decrease in recovery of [^{3}H]DPDPE-binding sites. However, a significant, though smaller, decrease in displaceable binding sites also occurred in the test with (D-Ala^2) deltorphin I (Fig. 2b).

An investigation of the ability of a variety of neuropeptides to displace specifically bound [^{3}H]DAMA in vertebrates as well as invertebrates (Stefano et al. 1992a) revealed that δ-opioid peptides are considerably more effective than μ- and κ-ligands.

Part of the difficulty of generating a binding isotherm with "standard" methods in the invertebrate species under consideration may be the low level of specific opioid binding in relation to the total number of heterogeneous hemocytes examined in invertebrates (Stefano, unpublished).

Since current information on opioid binding in invertebrate immunocytes is still so limited, a brief reference to comparable studies in nervous tissue (Leung and Stefano 1987; Stefano 1982) may serve to suggest that the degree of complexity resembles that found in vertebrate systems. These studies demonstrate the presence of at least two types of opiate/opioid-binding sites in invertebrates: high-affinity sites following the law of mass action and low-affinity sites characterized by markedly positive homotropic cooperativity (Kream et al. 1980). Reversibility of opioid binding in *Mytilus* nervous tissue was demonstrated by kinetic analyses (Kream et al. 1980). Tests to determine the ability of various ligands to displace specifically bound ^{125}I-labeled FK 33–824 had the following results: the opioid peptides tested (β-endorphin > FK 33–824 > DAMA) were the most potent, the opiate narcotics (etorphine > morphine > levorphanol) exhibited intermediate potencies, and the benzomorphans (cyclazocine > pentazocine) were the least potent. Dextrorphan (10 μM), the inactive enantiomer of levorphanol, did not compete for ^{125}I-labeled FK 33–824 binding (Kream et al. 1980; Stefano 1980). Opioid agonist binding in invertebrate neural tissue, as in that of vertebrates, is inhibited by sodium, whereas antagonist binding is enhanced (Stefano 1980).

Discussion

In addition to the problems discussed above, future efforts to reach a better understanding of opioid-induced responses of vertebrate as well as invertebrate immunocytes must take into account variability based on differences in the material examined. The limited data available thus far come from the examination of different types of immunocytes taken from different animals and animal species. Cellular responses may depend on age, functional states, and the time of year in which the experiments are performed (Stefano et al. 1989a, b; Scharrer and Stefano, this volume).

Signals targeted to immunoreactive cells as well as other cell types addressed by blood-borne messengers require highly sensitive receptors. The mobile character of immune cells demands frequent adjustments to constant changes in the immediate environment. The wide variety of the available types of signal molecules (neuropeptides, cytokines, etc.; see Smith, and Hughes and Chin, both in this volume) may permit the fine-tuning of cellular interactions required.

Recent results obtained with (D-Ala^2) deltorphin I provide additional support for the concept, based on earlier studies (Stefano et al. 1989a, b), that a special δ subtype of opioid receptor for immunoregulating Met-enkephalin exists on human granulocytes and their counterpart in invertebrates (Figs. 1, 2). This opioid, which has not been demonstrated in the immune system, shares with DAMA the high potency of its effect on immunocyte stimulation and its differential response to preincubation with DALCE (Figs. 1c, 2b). This suggests that these two compounds interact with the same binding sites. Therefore, the special opioid receptor postulated to mediate the effects of Met-enkephalin on immune function can be tentatively classified as a subtype, δ_2, of the classical δ receptor, δ_1.

As to the functional significance of this putative subtype of δ receptor, it is proposed to be dynamically associated with neutral endopeptidase 24.11 (NEP;

CD10, "enkephalinase;" Stefano et al. 1992b). This view is supported by the extremely low binding site density for [^{3}H](D-Ala^{2}) deltorphin I and [^{3}H]DAMA in these immunocytes. The low density of this receptor and the high fidelity of signal recognition regulated by NEP, may be considered to be advantages in accommodating additional signal molecules controlling these immunoactive cells.

The close hypothetical association of immunocyte neuropeptide receptors with NEP can be noted in a recent report by Shipp et al. (1991). These characteristics of granulocyte recognition and subsequent activation are critical for this cell since many different peptidergic signals have the potential to impact on each individual cell.

Conclusions

In evaluating the binding data available to date, one is left with the impression that the analysis of immunocyte receptors is still preliminary. What has become apparent is that the special requirements of an effective signaling system among immunoactive cells and between the immune system and the neuroendocrine system appear to be met by a rather complex mechanism. Readily adjustable fine-tuned responses are accomplished by multiple signal molecules and their corresponding receptors, individually working at specific concentrations (see also Scharrer and Stefano, this volume). The efficiency of the system makes possible psychoneuroimmunological interactions in man and comparable phenomena in animals (Smith and Blalock 1981). What the variability in the data available thus far indicates is that a hierarchy of modulatory mechanisms control individual spheres of activity. Each sphere of influence appears to have its own operating parameters, as noted in recent studies by Smith et al. (1992) and Duvaux-Miret et al. (1992).

Both the invertebrate and vertebrate data presented imply that the proportion of cells that have the potential to respond to the specific opioid challenges is rather small. The *Mytilus* data indicate that the shift from an inactive to an active state can occur rapidly, depending on previous stimulations or the state of the stimulating environment. Furthermore, it would seem that the number of opioid receptors per cell is small based on the presumed existence of immunocyte population subsets noted in earlier reports (Stefano et al. 1989a, b; Scharrer 1991) and supported by the studies of Hughes et al. (1990). It is of interest that this system appears to have been conserved in the course of a long evolutionary history (Stefano 1991).

Acknowledgements. The author wishes to thank collaborators and students who worked on various projects outlined in this chapter. The author's research was partially supported by DA-47392, NIMH-COR 17138, NSF INT-8803664, The Long Island Community Foundation, Inc., Hoffmann LaRoche Pharmaceuticals, The Upjohn Company, and the State University of New York Research Foundation.

References

Ausciello CM, Roda LG (1984) Leu-enkephalin binding to cultured human T-lymphocytes. Cell Biol Int Rep 8:353–362

Blalock JE (1989) A molecular basis for bidirectional communication between the immune and neuroendocrine systems. Physiol Rev 69:1–32

Boogaerts MA, Vermylen J, Deckmyn H, Roelant C, Verwilghen RL, Jacob HS, Moldow CF (1983) Enkephalins modify granulocyte-endothelial interactions by stimulating prostacyclin production. Thromb Haemost 50:572–576

Bowen WD, Hellewell SB, Kelemen M, Huey R, Stewart D (1987) Affinity labelling of δ-opiate receptors using [D-Ala^2, Leu^5, Cys^6]enkephalin. J Biol Chem 262:13434–13439

Brown SL, Tokuda S, Saland LC, Van Epps DE (1986) Opioid peptides: effects on leukocyte migration. In: Plotnikoff NP, Faith RE, Murgo AJ, Good R (eds) Enkephalins and endorphins stress and the immune system. Plenum, New York, pp 367–386

Carr DJJ, Kin CH, De Costa B, Jacobson AE, Rice KC, Blalock JE (1988a) Evidence for a δ-class opioid receptor on cells of the immune system. Cel Immunol 116:44–51

Carr DJJ, Bubien JK, Woods WT, Blalock JE (1988b) Opioid receptors on murine splenocytes. Ann NY Acad Sci 450:694–697

Casale TB, Bowman S, Kaliner M (1984) Induction of human cutaneous mast cell degranulation by opiates and endogenous opioid peptides: evidence for opiate and nonopiate receptor participation. J Allergy Clin Immunol 73:775–781

De Carolis C, De Sanctis G, Perricone R, Fraioli F, Fontana L (1984) Evidence for an inhibitory role of β-endorphin and other opioids on human total T rosette formation. Experientia 40: 738–740

Duvaux-Miret O, Stefano GB, Smith EM, Dissous C, Capron A (1992) Immunosuppression in the definitive and intermediate hosts of the human parasite Schistosoma mansoni by release of immunoactive neuropeptides. Proc Natl Acad Sci USA 89:778–781

Erspamer V, Melchiorri P, Falconieri-Erspamer G, Negri L, Corsi R, Severini C, Barra D, Simmaco M, Kreil G (1990) Deltorphins: a family of naturally occurring peptides with high affinity and selectivity for δ opioid binding sites. Proc Natl Acad Sci USA 86:5188–5192

Faith RE, Liang HJ, Murgo AJ, Plotnikoff NP (1984) Neuroimmunomodulation with enkephalins: enhancement of human natural killer (NK) cell activity in vitro. Clin Immunol Immunopathol 31:412–418

Falke NE, Fischer EG (1985) Cell shape of polymorphonuclear leukocytes is influenced by opioids. Immunobiology 169:532–539

Falke NE, Fischer EG (1986) Opiate receptor mediated internalization of ^{125}I-β-endorphin in human polymorphonuclear leucocytes. Cell Biol Int Rep 10:429–437

Farrar WL (1984) Endorphin modulation of lymphokine activity. In: Fraiolo F, Isidori A, Mazzetti M (eds) Opioid peptides in the periphery. Elsevier, Amsterdam, pp 159–167

Fjellner B, Hagermark O (1982) Potentiation of histamine-induced itch and flare responses in human skin by the enkephalin analogue FK 33–824, β-endorphin and morphine. Arch Dermatol Res 274:29–35

Foris G, Medgyesi GA, Gyimesi E, Hauck M (1984) Met-enkephalin induced alterations of macrophage functions. Mol Immunol 21:747–754

Foris G, Medgyesi GA, Hauck M (1986) Bidirectional effect of Met-enkephalin on macrophage effector functions. Mol Cell Biochem 69:127–134

Froelich CJ, Bankhurst AD (1984) The effect of β-endorphin on natural cytotoxicity and antibody dependent cellular cytotoxicity. Life Sci 35:261–269

Gilman SC, Schwartz JM, Milner RJ, Bloom FE, Feldman JD (1982) β-Endorphin enhances lymphocyte proliferative responses. Proc Natl Acad Sci USA 79:4226–4230

Hazum E, Chang KJ, Cuatrecasas P (1979) Specific nonopiate receptors for β-endorphin. Science 205:1033–1035

Heijnen CJ, Bevers C, Kavelaars A, Ballieux RE (1986) Effect of β-endorphin on the antigen-induced primary antibody response of human blood B cells in vitro. J Immunol 136:213–218

Hughes TK Jr, Smith EM, Chin R, Cadet P, Sinisterra J, Leung MK, Shipp MA, Scharrer B, Stefano GB (1990) Interaction of immunoactive monokines (IL-1 and TNF) in the bivalve mollusc Mytilus edulis. Proc Natl Acad Sci USA 87:4426–4429

Janković BD, Marić D (1988) Enkephalins modulate in vivo immune reactions through δ- and μ-opioid receptors. Ann NY Acad Sci 450:691–693

Johnson HM, Smith EM, Torres BA, Blalock JE (1982) Regulation of the in vitro antibody response by neuroendocrine hormones. Proc Natl Acad Sci USA 79:4171–4174

Kay M, Allen J, Morley JE (1984) Endorphins stimulate normal human peripheral blood lymphocyte natural killer activity. Life Sci 35:53–58

Kream RM, Zukin RS, Stefano GB (1980) Demonstration of two classes of opiate binding sites in the nervous tissue of the marine mollusc Mytilus edulis: positive homotropic cooperativity of lower affinity binding sites. J Biol Chem 225(19):9218–9224

Leung MK, Stefano GB (1987) Comparative neurobiology of opioids in invertebrates with special attention to senescent alterations. Prog Neurobiol 28:131–159

Liu JS, Garrett KM, Lin SCC, Way EL (1983) The effects of opiates on calcium accumulation on rat peritoneal mast cells. Eur J Pharmacol 91:335–341

Lopker A, Abood LG, Hoss W, Lionetti FJ (1980) Stereoselective muscarinic acetylcholine and opiate receptors in human phagocytic leukocytes. Biochem Pharmacol 29:1361–1365

Mandler RN, Biddison WE, Mandler R, Serrate SA (1986) β-endorphin augments the cytolytic activity and interferon production of natural killer cells. J Immunol 136:934–935

Marić D, Janković BD (1988) Suppression of anaphylactic shock by enkephalins. Ann NY Acad Sci 450:684–687

Mathews PM, Froelich CJ, Sibbitt WL Jr, Bankhurst AD (1983) Enhancement of natural cytotoxicity by β-endorphin. J Immunol 130:1658–1662

McCain HW, Lamster I, Bozzone JM, Grbic JT (1982) β-Endorphin modulates human immune activity via non-opiate receptor mechanisms. Life Sci 31:1619–1624

Mehrishi JN, Mills IH (1983) Opiate receptors on lymphocytes and platelets in man. Clin Immunol Immunopathol 27:240–249

Miller GC, Murgo AJ, Plotnikoff NP (1983) Enkephalins-enhancement of active T-cell rosettes from lymphoma patients. Clin Immunol Immunopathol 26:446–451

Miller GC, Murgo AJ, Plotnikoff NP (1984) Enkephalins-enhancement of active T-cell rosettes from normal volunteers. Clin Immunol Immunopathol 31:132–136

Plotnikoff NP, Miller GC (1983) Enkephalins as immunomodulators. Int J Immunopharmacol 5: 437–441

Radulescu RT, DeCosta BR, Jacobson AE, Rice KC, Blalock JE, Carr DJJ (1991) Biochemical and functional characterization of a μ-opioid receptor binding site on cells of the immune system. Prog Neuroendocrinimmunol 4:166–179

Sharp BM, Keane WF, Suh HJ, Gekker G, Tsukayama D, Peterson PK (1985) Opioid peptides rapidly stimulate superoxide production by human polymorphonuclear leukocytes and macrophages. Endocrinology 117:793–799

Scharrer B (1991) Neuroimmunology: the importance and role of a comparative approach. Adv Neuroimmunol 1:1–16

Shavit Y, Lewis JW, Terman GW, Gale RP, Liebeskind JC (1984) Opioid peptides mediate the suppressive effect of stress on natural killer cell cytotoxicity. Science 223:188–190

Shavit Y, Terman GW, Martin FC, Lewis JW, Liebeskind JC, Gale RP (1985) Stress, opioid peptides, the immune system, and cancer. J Immunol 135s:834–838

Shavit Y, Terman GW, Lewis JW, Zane CJ, Gale RP, Liebeskind JC (1986) Effects of footshock stress and morphine on natural killer lymphocytes in rats: studies of tolerance and cross-tolerance. Brain Res 372:382–387

Shipp MA, Stefano GB, D'Adamio L, Switzer SN, Howard FD, Sinisterra J, Scharrer B, Reinherz E (1990) CD10/Neutral endopeptidase 24.11 ("enkephalinase") downregulates enkephalin-mediated inflammatory responses in invertebrate and mammalian organisms. Nature 347: 394–396

Shipp MA, Stefano GB, Switzer SN, Griffin JD, Reinherz EL (1991) CD10 (CALLA)/neutral endopeptidase 24.11 modulates inflammatory peptide-induced changes in neutrophil morphology, migration, and adhesion proteins and is itself regulated by neutrophil activation. Blood 78:1834–1841

Sibinga NES, Goldstein A (1988) Opioid peptides and opioid receptors in cells of the immune system. Annu Rev Immunol 6:219–249

Smith EM, Blalock JE (1981) Human lymphocyte production of corticotropin and endorphin-like substances: association with leukocyte interferon. Proc Natl Acad Sci USA 78:7530–7535

Smith EM, Hughes TK, Hashemi F, Stefano GB (1992) Immunosuppressive effects of ACTH and MSH and their possible significance in human immunodeficiency virus infection. Proc Natl Acad Sci USA 89:782–786

Stefano GB (1980) Opiates and neuroactive pentapeptides: binding characteristics and interactions with dopamine stimulated adenylate cyclase in the pedal ganglia of Mytilus edulis. Adv Physiol Sci 22:423–453

Stefano GB (1982) Comparative aspects of opioid-dopamine interaction. Cell Mol Neurobiol 2:167–178

Stefano GB (1989) Role of opioid neuropeptides in immunoregulation. Prog Neurobiol 33:149–159

Stefano GB (1991) Conformational matching a stabilizing signal system factor during evolution: additional evidence in comparative neuroimmunology. Adv Neuroimmunol 1:71–82

Stefano GB, Leung MK, Zhao X, Scharrer B (1989a) Evidence for the involvement of opioid neuropeptides in the adherence and migration of immunocompetent invertebrate hemocytes. Proc Natl Acad Sci USA 86:626–630

Stefano GB, Cadet P, Scharrer B (1989b) Stimulatory effects of opioid neuropeptides on locomotory activity and conformational changes in invertebrate and human immunocytes: evidence for a subtype of δ receptor. Proc Natl Acad Sci USA 86:6307–6311

Stefano GB, Melchiorri P, Hughes TK, Scharrer B (1992a) Deltorphin I binding and pharmacological evidence for a novel subtype of δ-opioid receptor on human and invertebrate immune cells. Proc Natl Acad Sci USA 89:9316–9320

Stefano GB, Paemen LR, Hughes TK (1992b) Modulation of CD10/neutral endopeptidase 24.11 by tumor necrosis factor and neuropeptides in immunocytes: implications in autoimmunomodulation. J Neuroimmunol 41:9–14

Wybran J (1985) Enkephalins and endorphins: activation molecules for the immune system and natural killer activity? Neuropeptides 5:371–377

Wybran J, Appelboom T, Famaey JP, Govaerts A (1979) Suggestive evidence for receptors for morphine and methionine-enkephalin on normal human blood T lymphocytes. J Immunol 123: 1068–1070

Yamasaki Y, Shimamura O, Kizu A, Nakagawa N, Ijichi H (1983) Interactions of morphine with PGE1, isoproterenol, dopamine, and aminophylline in rat mast cells; their effect on IgE-mediated ^{14}C-serotonin release. Agents Actions 13:21–27

Degradation of Neuropeptide Signal Molecules in Immunocytes of Vertebrates and Invertebrates

A. J. Turner[1], M. K. Leung[2], and G. B. Stefano[2]

Introduction

There are now substantial grounds for believing that the enkephalins have multiple physiological roles and can serve as neurotransmitters, neurohormones, or neuromodulators as well as immunomodulators. Other neuropeptides also function as signaling molecules in both the nervous and immune systems. It is therefore important to establish the mechanism by which the peptide signal is terminated. Previous studies (see, for example Turner et al. 1987) have ruled out a presynaptic uptake mechanism for neuropeptides in general. It has been demonstrated that if enkephalin is added to neural tissues or blood, it is rapidly metabolized (Lane et al. 1977; Vogel and Altstein 1979). This fact alone does not demonstrate the presence of a specific "enkephalinase." Indeed, a nonspecific enzyme may serve equally well since specificity may be achieved by the location of the enzyme and the presence of only enkephalinergic signal molecules. The consensus of opinion now is that specific "neuropeptidases" do not exist, but rather that a handful of enzymes located at the cell surface of many different cell types can act in concert to degrade regulatory peptides. To date there is only one exception to this general rule: pyroglutamyl aminopeptidase II (EC 3.4.19.-), a metalloenzyme which appears to be a specific degrading enzyme for thyrotropin-releasing hormone (Wilk 1986). Much of our understanding of neuropeptide metabolism has come from a study of the peptidases of the mammalian renal brush-border membrane. This membrane preparation represents an abundant source of peptidases which are also expressed, at lower levels, in the nervous and immune systems. A description of these activities provides a useful foreword to a discussion of immunocyte peptidases. A more detailed review of brush-border peptidases can be found in Turner (1987) and Kenny and Turner (1987).

[1]Department of Biochemistry and Molecular Biology, The University of Leeds, Leeds, LS2 9JT, UK
[2]Multidisciplinary Center for the Study of Aging, Old Westbury Neuroscience Research Institute, State University of New York, College at Old Westbury, Old Westbury, NY 11568, USA

Scharrer et al. (Eds.)
Neuropeptides and Immunoregulation

Brush-Border Membrane Peptidases

Microvilli, especially those located in the proximal convoluted tubule of the kidney, are abundant in peptidases. Simple preparative methods for isolation of microvilli provide a ready source for characterization of these enzymes. Table 1 lists the main peptidases located in renal microvilli. Most species contain only a single endopeptidase (endopeptidase 24.11; neutral endopeptidase, NEP) although rodent species contain a second endopeptidase referred to as endopeptidase-2 (rat) or meprin (mouse). Since many regulatory peptides are blocked at N- or C-termini, their hydrolysis must be initiated by endopeptidase action, hence the central role that NEP has assumed in studies of peptide degradation. The action of this enzyme can then be complemented by exopeptidases such as aminopeptidases or carboxypeptidases. All of these enzymes have the topology of ectoenzymes (Fig. 1), i.e., they are integral plasma membrane proteins in which the bulk of the enzyme, including the catalytic domain, faces the extracellular space. They are therefore ideally situated to terminate the peptidergic signal. This is especially true for the opioid immuno-responsive immunocyte of invertebrates and human polymorphonuclear leukocyte (Shipp et al. 1990). Nearly all the peptidases in the brush-border are metalloenzymes, with zinc usually being identified as the catalytic metal ion. Dipeptidyl peptidase IV is an exception in being a serine enzyme.

Endopeptidase 24.11

NEP was originally identified as a renal membrane enzyme that hydrolyzes the B chain of insulin. Subsequent characterization (Kerr and Kenny 1974) revealed the enzyme to have a broad specificity, hydrolysing on the amino side of a hydrophobic amino acid residue. In this respect NEP closely resembles thermolysin although there are some subsite differences in specificity (Hersh and Morihara 1986). The enzyme was subsequently "rediscovered" to be involved in the hydrolysis of the Gly^3-Phe^4 bond of the enkephalins in the brain and hence was also termed "enkephalinase" (Malfroy et al. 1978). More detailed studies have revealed the enzyme to be widely distributed but not ubiquitous in mammalian tissues (Gee et al. 1985). It is present on other brush-borders (intestine, placenta, and choroid plexus), reticular cells in the lymph nodes (Bowes and Kenny 1986), neutrophils (Painter et al. 1988), as well as some endocrine cells (Kenny et al. 1987). It is absent in normal lymphocytes, liver, and muscle. In the central nervous system it is localized to neuronal membranes (Barnes et al. 1988) where it probably plays a role in inactivating tachykinins such as substance P as well as the enkephalins (Matsas et al. 1983). Another major role for the enzyme is in the inactivation of atrial and brain natriuretic peptides (Stephenson and Kenny 1987; Vogt-Schaden et al. 1989; Medeiros et al. 1991),

Table 1. The major membrane peptidases of the kidney brush-border

Enzyme	Subunit M_r ($\times 10^{-3}$)	Specificity	Active site	cDNA sequence available	Topology	Synonyms
Endopeptidase-24.11	90–100	–○–○–↓●–○–○– (hydrophobic)	Zn^{2+}	Yes	N-in/C-out	Neutral endopeptidase; enkephalinase; atriopeptidase; CALLA; CD-10
Endopeptidase-2 (rat)	80 + 74	–○–○–↓/↓●–○–○– (aromatic)	Zn^{2+}	Yes	C-in/N-out	Meprin (mouse); endopeptidase-24.18
Angiotensin-converting enzyme	180	–○–○–↓●–● (nonspecific)	Zn^{2+}	Yes	C-in/N-out	Peptidyl dipeptidase A; kininase II
Aminopeptidase N	150–160	●↓–○–○–○– (nonspecific)	Zn^{2+}	Yes	N-in/C-out	Aminopeptidase M; CD13; gp150
Aminopeptidase A	170	●↓–○–○–○– (Glu/Asp)	Ca^{2+}(?)	Yes	N-in/C-out	BP-1/6C3
Aminopeptidase P	94	○–↓●–○–○– (Pro)	Zn^{2+}	No	GPI	

Aminopeptidase W	130	○-↓●-○-○- (Trp)	Zn^{2+}	No	?	
Carboxypeptidase M	62	-○-○-○-↓● (Arg/Lys)	Zn^{2+} (?)	Yes	GPI	
Carboxypeptidase P	135	-○-○-●-↓○ (Pro)	Zn^{2+}	No	?	
Dipeptidyl peptidase IV	110–130	○-●-↓○-○- (Pro/Ala)	Ser	Yes	N-in/C-out	CD26; gp100; THAM
Membrane dipeptidase	47	●-↓● (nonspecific)	Zn^{2+}	Yes	GPI	Renal or microsomal dipeptidase; dehydropeptidase I
γ-Glutamyl transpeptidase	60 + 30	●-↓○-○- (γ-Glu)		Yes	N-in/C-out	γ-Glutamyltransferase

All the enzymes listed are integral membrane proteins existing as ectoenzymes, N-in/C-out indicates the N-terminus is cytosolic with the C-terminus extracellular; the converse applies for C-in/N-out. GPI indicates a glycosyl-phosphatidylinositol membrane anchor.

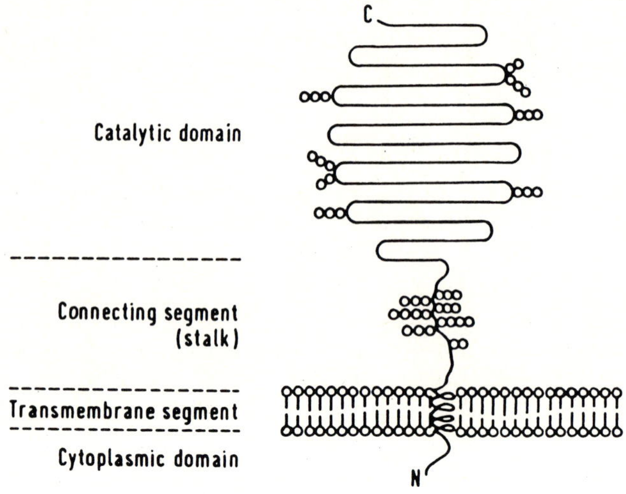

Fig. 1. Topology of N-terminally anchored (N-in/C-out) ectoenzyme such as endopeptidase-24.11 or aminopeptidase N

and inhibitors of NEP are undergoing intensive evaluation as anti-hypertensive agents (see for example, Roques and Beaumont 1990). In the peripheral nervous system NEP is located on some Schwann cell membranes, where its function is unknown (Matsas et al. 1986). The following list summarizes the tissue distribution of NEP in the pig:

Epithelia
- Brush-border (kidney, intestine, placenta, choroid plexus)
- Cells lining reproductive tract (male and female)

Myoepithelia
- Salivary glands
- Sweat glands
- Rectal glands

Connective tissue
- Reticular cell (lymph nodes)
- Chondrocytes (articular cartilage)

Endocrine cells
- Steroid: zona glomerulosa, Leydig cells (testis), interstitial cells (ovary)
- Peptide: pituitary gonadotrophs

Central nervous system
- Some neuronal membranes

Peripheral nervous system
- Schwann cell membranes

Peripheral blood
Polymorphonuclear leukocytes
Pre B-cells (bone marrow)
CALLA$^+$ cells

NEP has a distinct preference for relatively small peptides (typically up to 30 residues) as substrate, and these substrates may be neurotransmitters, neuromodulators, or peptide hormones. Much less is known of the species distribution and evolution of NEP. It has been studied in detail in several mammalian species, but an NEP-like activity has been detected in the electric organ of *Torpedo marmorata* (Turner and Dowdall 1984), in synaptic membranes from the locust *Schistocerca gregaria* (Isaac 1988), and more recently in some other invertebrate species such as the mollusc *Mytilus edulis* (Shipp et al. 1990). The usual criterion for identification as NEP is its substrate specificity, particularly its ability to hydrolyse the Gly-Phe bond in [Met^5]-and [Leu^5]-enkephalins, coupled with sensitivity to inhibition by phosphoramidon or thiorphan (see, for example, Turner 1987). However, at least one other phosphoramidon-sensitive endopeptidase is known in mammalian cells (endothelin-converting enzyme, Hioki et al. 1991), and inhibition data alone are not sufficient for identification as NEP. In the case of the *M. edulis* enkephalin-degrading activity (Shipp et al. 1990) cross-reactivity with an antiserum to human NEP supports identity with mammalian NEP and suggests considerable preservation of NEP structure through evolution.

NEP Identical with the Common Acute Lymphoblastic Leukemia Antigen

Molecular cloning of NEP has confirmed its identity as an ectoenzyme (Fig. 1; Devault et al. 1987; Malfroy et al. 1987). The structure is consistent with that originally predicted from protein chemical studies (Fulcher et al. 1986) with a short N-terminal cytoplasmic domain (of 20–30 amino acids depending on species) followed by a stretch of 23 predominantly hydrophobic amino acids which comprise the membrane anchor which represents the uncleaved signal peptide (Malfroy et al. 1987; Devault et al. 1987). The bulk of the protein, including the active site, is then located extracellularly. The enzyme contains the characteristic "zinc signature" (His-Glu-Xaa-His; Jongeneel et al. 1989) as befits a zinc metallopeptidase. Subsequently, molecular cloning and sequencing of the common acute lymphoblastic leukemia antigen (CALLA; CD-10) revealed it to be virtually identical with the predicted sequence of NEP (LeTarte et al. 1988; Shipp et al. 1988, 1989). CALLA is a 100-kDa tumor-associated glycoprotein antigen. It was first described by Greaves et al. (1975) and is expressed on lymphoblasts from most (>90%) patients with the common type of acute lymphoblastic leukemia and on cells from patients with chronic myelocytic leukemia in lymphoid blast crisis and other lymphoid malignancies with an immature phenotype (Brown et al. 1975; Ritz et al. 1980; Greaves et al. 1983). it is also expressed by terminally differentiated polymorphonuclear leukocytes (Cossmann et al. 1983) and on human gliomas (Carrel et al. 1982) and in malignant melanoma (Carrel et al. 1983). Antibodies against CALLA have been used extensively in the diagnosis and therapy of lymphoid malignancies. Although originally thought to be a tumor-specific antigen, CALLA was subsequently reported on some non-hematopoietic cell types and was shown to be abundant in kidney and intestine (Tredosiewicz et al. 1985). Until the identity of NEP and CALLA was noted (LeTarte et al. 1988), no activity had been described for the antigen which had been identified solely by immunological criteria. The cDNA sequences of CALLA/NEP have now been determined from four tissue sources (leukemia cells, kidney, brain, and placenta) in three species (human, rabbit, and rat; Devault et al. 1987; Malfroy et al. 1987, 1988; LeTarte et al. 1988; Shipp et al. 1988). Transfection of a non-CD10-containing cell line with CD10 resulted in cell surface NEP enzymatic activity, confirming the functional identity of CD10/CALLA with NEP (Shipp et al. 1989).

In retrospect, the possible identities of NEP and CALLA/CD10 might have been predicted earlier purely on the basis of their tissue distributions and physicochemical properties. It had already been established that NEP is located on reticular cells in the pig lymph nodes although it is absent from normal lymphocytes (Bowes and Kenny 1986). Its presence in the immune system had already prompted speculation on a role in the inactivation of immune mediators (Kenny et al. 1987). In support of this hypothesis, Pierart et al. (1988) have shown that interleukin-1 (IL-1) activity in a thymocyte proliferation assay disappeared on incubation with purified NEP, and this inactivation was prevented by the NEP inhibitor phosphoramidon. Slow degradation of IL-1β was detected when it was exposed to purified NEP (Stefano, unpublished data). More recent studies have, however, failed to support a role for NEP in IL-1 degradation in vivo (Poole et al. 1990), making it likely that other immunoregulatory peptides are the targets for NEP in the immune system.

A strong candidate for such an NEP substrate is thymic humoral factor γ_2, which is a small immunoregulatory peptide present in thymic extracts recently identified as the octapeptide Leu-Glu-Asp-Gly-Pro-Lys-Phe-Leu (Burstein et al. 1988). Bovine kidney NEP was shown to hydrolyze thymic humoral factor γ_2 efficiently at the Lys-Phe bond with a similar K_m and k_{cat} as for the hydrolysis of Leu-enkephalin (Indig et al. 1991). Intriguingly, the C-terminal dipeptide of the thymic peptide (Phe-Leu) is identical with that in the enkephalins, which presumably explains the comparable efficiencies of hydrolysis. The purified thymic factor has been shown to augment multiple T-cell functions and to stimulate production of IL-2. Inhibitors of NEP may therefore be of benefit in augmenting responses to such immunoregulatory peptides.

Invertebrate NEP Homolog: Specificity and Functional Studies

Some general aspects of mammalian NEP specificity have been defined (Table 2). In a summary chart Turner et al. (1985) listed the "best" to the "worst" peptide substrates [substance P > Met-enkephalin-Arg^6-Phe^7 > physalaemin > bradykinin > DAla^2-Leu^5 enkephalin > Leu-enkephalin > Met-enkephalin > CCK-8- > dynorphin > neurotensin > D-Ala^2-Met^5 enkephalin (DAMA) > D-Ala^2-Leu^5-enkephalinamide]. It is important to note from the perspective of several studies (Stefano et al. 1989a,b, 1991; Shipp et al. 1990) that, although neutral endopeptidase can cleave DAMA, its preferential activity in this regard is quite low. Additionally, it was demonstrated that Met-enkephalin-Arg^6-Phe^7 degradation and subsequent loss of stimulating activity can be prevented by concomitant treatment with the NEP inhibitor phosphoramidon in vitro for both immunoreactive invertebrate immunocytes and human polymorphonuclear leukocytes (Stefano et al. 1990). Additionally, DAMA appears to be less susceptible to NEP action in cell stimulatory bioassays as compared to Met-enkephalin and the opioid heptapeptide (Shipp et al. 1990; Stefano et al. 1990). These data agree with the rank order of preference of NEP in the review by Turner et al. (1985). This agreement underscores the potential significance of this enzyme in these diverse animal phyla, especially given the striking parallels in the modulation of immunopeptidergic signals. Clearly, its localization on the membrane of these "blood" cells, most probably in the vicinity of respective peptidergic receptors, further suggests an important role in the termination of action of the peptidergic signal molecules as well as the modulation of local "environmental" levels of the respective signal molecules. It certainly aids in the understanding of why Met-enkephalin is normally not as potent as DAMA in inducing conformational alterations of immunocytes associated with "activation."

The role of Met-enkephalin in mediating invertebrate inflammatory responses (Stefano et al. 1989a,b) prompted an investigation to determine whether invertebrate organisms, such as *M. edulis* express a CD10/NEP homolog. Recent studies indicate that Met-enkephalin, which is present in the hemolymph of invertebrate organisms, stimulates hemocytes to flatten, develop pseudopodia, and undergo directed migration and formation of cell clusters (Stefano et al. 1989a,b). These Met-enkephalin mediated effects are inhibited by naloxone, indicating that they result from the specific interaction of the neuropeptide with its opioid receptor (Stefano et al. 1989a,b).

To determine whether *M. edulis* hemocytes express a CD10/NEP homolog hemocytes were analyzed for cell surface CD10 enzymatic activity by use of a sensitive fluorimetric assay (Shipp et al. 1989, 1990). It was found that *M. edulis* hemocytes have readily detectable functional CD10/NEP activity (approximately 3000 nmol/h per 10^6 cell) that is reduced by the specific NEP inhibitor phosphoramidon (Matsas et al. 1984; Shipp et al. 1990) The identity of invertebrate NEP was confirmed with hemocyte lysates that were size-fractionated, blotted, and probed with a heteroantiserum (anti-hu-CD10) raised against denatured,

Table 2. Hydrolysis of opioid peptides by endopeptidase-24.11 (from Turner et al. 1987)

Peptide	Sites of hydrolysis	$k_m (\mu M)$	k_{cat} (min^{-1})	k_{cat}/K_m (min^{-1} μM^{-1})
[Leu[5]] enkephalin	Y G G↓F L	86	3781	43.9
[D-Ala[2], Leu[5]] enkephalin	YdA G↓F L	88	5645	64.2
[Leu[5]] enkephalinamide	Y G G↓F L NH_2	680	1129	1.7
[D-Ala[2], Leu[5]] enkephalinamide	YdA G↓F L NH_2	773	1659	2.1
Dynorphin-(1–9)-peptide	Y G G⇣F⇣L R R↓I R	219	5340	24.4
[Met[5]] enkephalin	Y G G↓F M	62	2597	41.9
[D-Ala[2], Met[5]] enkephalinamide	YdA G↓F M NH_2	432	6132	14.2
[Met[5]] enkephalin-Arg[6]	Y G G↓F M R	38	2062	53.6
[Met[5]] enkephalin-Arg[6]-Phe[7]	Y G G↓F M R	50	5198	117.4
		$K_i (\mu M)$	V_{max} (relative to [Leu[5]] enkephalin	
β-Lipotropin-(61–69)-peptide	Y G G↓F M T S E K	19	0.44	
α-Neo-endorphin	Y G G↓F L R K Y P K	>500		
β-Neo-endorphin	Y G G↓F L R K Y P	>500		
Dynorphin-(1–13)-peptide	Y G G↓F L R R⇣I R P K⇣L K	>500		
γ-Endorphin	Y G G⇣F M T S E K S Q T P↓L V T L	42	0.92	
β-Endorphin	Y G G↓F M T S E K S Q T P⇣L V T L- F K N A I↓I K N A⇣Y K K G E	>500		

gel-purified human CD10 protein (Shipp et al. 1990). The results of this determination were positive (Shipp et al. 1990). Thus, the immunoreactivity and enzymatic assays indicate that *M. edulis* hemocytes express a functional CD10/NEP related structure (Shipp et al. 1990).

To determine whether the putative invertebrate CD10/NEP regulates local Met-enkephalin levels and thereby modulates enkephalin-mediated changes as noted above, *M. edulis* hemocytes were stimulated in vitro with Met-enkephalin at 10^{-6}–10^{-12} *M* in the presence or absence of NEP inhibitors (Shipp et al. 1990). As reported (Shipp et al. 1990), phosphoramidon reduces the minimum concentration of Met-enkephalin required to trigger morphological hemocyte changes and increases in cell area by five orders of magnitude. Captopril, which inhibits peptidyldipeptidase A (angiotensin-converting enzyme, ACE), but is inactive against NEP (Matsas et al. 1984), had no effect on Metenkephalin triggered hemocyte activation. The same experiments were repeated with human polymorphonuclear leukocytes, yielding similar results. These data suggest that CD10/NEP regulates local Met-enkephalin levels and resultant enkephalin-mediated immune responses in organisms that are 500 million years divergent in evolution (Meglitsch 1967). The previously noted heterogeneity in Met-enkephalin effects may be related to variable CD10/NEP expression (Van Epps and Saland 1984; Fischer and Falke 1987; Van Epps and Kutvirt 1987). The regulation of this neuropeptide signal via coexpression of cell surface receptors and the CD10/NEP hydrolytic enzyme resembles the cholinergic signal system, where both acetylcholine receptors and acetylcholinesterase are in operation (Raftery et al. 1980; Massoulie and Bon 1982). The potentiation of cholinergic stimulation by inhibition of acetylcholinesterase resembles the Met-enkephalin phenomenon described by Shipp et al. (1990). However, Erdös et al. (1989) demonstrated that CD10/NEP is rapidly downregulated and internalized when human polymorphonuclear leukocytes are stimulated with either phorbol myristate acetate or a diacylglycerol analog. This suggests that, in addition to regulating local neuropeptide levels, CD10/NEP is itself affected by the activation state of the target cell.

Aminopeptidase(s)

The degradative enzymes reported to be present in peripheral fluids are aminopeptidase, endopeptidase, and carboxypeptidase. Moreover, exogenous enkephalins are degraded rapidly when added to mammalian serum or invertebrate hemolymph (Dupont et al. 1977; Hambrook et al. 1976; Leung and Lundy 1990). In this same report the major degradative product found after incubating Met-enkephalin with rat plasma was that of Tyr and Gly-Gly-Phe-Met, indicating that the main degradative enzyme in plasma is aminopeptidase. This is in agreement with an earlier study which indicates that the major enkephalin degrading enzyme in the plasma of mammals is aminopeptidase (Venturelli et al. 1985).

The presence of Gly-Gly-Phe-Met and Phe-Met in HPLC peaks of fractionated cell-free *M. edulis* hemolymph indicates the presence of aminopeptidase- and endopeptidase-like enzymes. Met-enkephalin is degraded mainly by aminopeptidase in the cell-free hemolymph fluid (Leung and Lundy 1990; Leung 1990). At 500 μ*M* the half-life of Met-enkephalin in mussel hemolymph is 9 min; in the presence of 100 μ*M* phosphoramidon the half-life is extended to 16 min. This clearly shows the presence of phosphoramidon inhibitable activity in the hemolymph fluid. The endopeptidase activity found in the cell-free hemolymph fluid probably came from membrane bound endopeptidase on hemocyte membrane fragments in the fluid (Shipp et al. 1990). Results from more recent studies with the use of debris-free hemolymph prepared by high-speed centrifugation and hemocyte membrane preparation showed that the cleavage of Met-enkephalin to Tyr-Gly-Gly and Phe-Met in the hemolymph fluid is inhibited by captopril while the same cleavage in the membrane preparation is inhibited by phosphoramidon (Leung, unpublished data). Thus, the cleavage of the Gly-Phe bond of Met-enkephalin is a consequence of the action of ACE in the hemolymph fluid and NEP on the hemocyte membrane. Even though ACE is generally considered to be membrane bound, a low level of ACE is found in mammalian serum.

The role of aminopeptidase in the degradation of Met-enkephalin is implicated by the enhancement of conformational change in hemocytes obtained from the mussel after injection of Met-enkephalin (1 n*M*) with bestatin (1 m*M*), a potent inhibitor of aminopeptidase. The number of "active-ameboid" hemocytes obtained from resting animals is approximately 6% of the harvested cells (Stefano et al. 1989a,b). Concomitant injection of Met-enkephalin with bestatin increased the number of active hemocytes obtained after 1 h to 17%, strongly indicating the presence of aminopeptidase. This result supports our previous conclusions that endogenous proteases are present in invertebrates, and that therefore unless appropriate measures are taken, it is difficult to demonstrate enkephalinergic activities (Leung and Stefano 1987).

Thus far enkephalin degradation in hemolymph has been examined in three invertebrate species. In the hemolymph of the crayfish *Astacus fluviatilis* and the horse shoe crab *Limulus polyphemus* similar degradation enzyme activities as those in *Mytilus edulis* were observed (Coletti-Previero et al. 1981). Differing from that in mammalian serum, the major activity found in the hemolymph of these two organisms is carboxypeptidase and not aminopeptidase. Two additional enkephalin degrading enzymes present in *Astacus* and *Limulus* hemolymph were found to have aminopeptidase and dipeptidylcarboxypeptidase activities. The total activity of these two enzymes was relatively small and represented only about 10% of all the degradative activities in the hemolymph. All three enzymes are inhibited by 1,10-phenanthroline and are therefore likely to belong to the zinc metalloprotease family. Interestingly, the dipeptidylcarboxypeptidase activity was not inhibited by phosphoramidon, suggesting that this enzyme is different from NEP.

Thus, it appears that even though the types of enkephalin degrading enzymes found in the circulating fluids of different organisms are similar, significant differences exist in terms of their relative activities. The levels of different enkephalin degrading enzyme activities found in *Mytilus* resemble those found in mammalian plasma rather than *Astacus* and *Limulus* hemolymph. Experiments carried out with cell-free hemolymph fluid demonstrated that the major enzyme activity in *Mytilus* hemolymph, as with human plasma, is aminopeptidase (Leung and Le 1991). The aminopeptidase activity is inhibited by amastatin and bestatin but not by phosphoramidon, thiorphan, captopril, or other ACE inhibitors (Leung, unpublished data). This suggests that the aminopeptidase found in *Mytilus* is similar to that in human plasma.

Additional Cell-Surface Peptidases Identical With Cluster Differentiation Antigens

The myeloid cell-surface glycoprotein antigen gp150 or CD13 is expressed on at least 70% of acute myeloid leukemia cells, and antibodies to this antigen are therefore important diagnostic reagents. Cloning and sequencing of CD13 revealed its identity as aminopeptidase N (Table 1) (Look et al. 1989). As with CALLA, CD13 shows a lineage-dependent expression and is found on myeloid progenitors, monocytes, granulocytes, and myeloid leukemia cells. In addition, it is abundantly expressed in the renal brush-border and intestine as well as other locations. Aminopeptidase N constitutes as much as 8% of the membrane protein in the renal brush-border. It is a zinc-containing integral membrane glycoprotein of subunit M_r 160,000 in the pig, although the native enzyme probably exists as a dimer in the membrane (Hussain et al. 1981). It exhibits a broad substrate specificity as an aminopeptidase with alanine as the most "favored" residue at the N-terminus. Small peptides with bulky hydrophobic amino acids at the N-terminus (e.g., Leu) are also good substrates, but leucinamide is not hydrolyzed. This distinguishes aminopeptidase N from the cytosolic "leucine aminopeptidase" with which it is often confused. Important physiological substrates for aminopeptidase N are the enkephalins, although at least one other membrane aminopeptidase is able to hydrolyze these opioid peptides (Matsas et al. 1985). The relation of these activities to the enkephalin aminopeptidase (s) in serum and hemolymph (see above) remains to be resolved. The role of aminopeptidase N on myeloid cells is unknown although it is conceivable that it may contribute to antigen processing on monocytes. Bestatin, an aminopeptidase N inhibitor, stimulates T- and B-cell responses in vivo and in vitro; however, whether this action is via aminopeptidase inhibition or some other effect is unclear.

An alveolar epithelial cell antigen, previously designated p146 and implicated in lung cell differentiation, has now also been identified as aminopeptidase N (Funkhouser et al. 1991). Partial amino acid sequencing of rat p146 was consistent with the aminopeptidase N sequence, and immunoaffinity-purified p146 displayed the appropriate enzymic activity. Thus, aminopeptidase N may play a role in lineage-dependent differentiation in a variety of cell types. A critical question to answer is the nature of the peptide substrate (s) in the vicinity of these cells.

Another cell-surface glycoprotein of interest is an antigen originally identified immunologically in mice by the monoclonal antibody BP-1 and by the rat monoclonal 6C3 (Cooper et al. 1986; Wu et al. 1989). The BP-1/6C3 antigen is expressed on early B-lineage cells in hematopoietic tissues but is not found on mature lymphocytes in peripheral lymphoid tissues. The glycoprotein has been postulated to play an important role in controlling the growth and differentiation of early B-lineage cells (Wu et al. 1990). These authors have isolated and sequenced cDNAs encoding the BP-1/6C3 antigen, and the cDNA sequence predicted a type II integral membrane protein of 945 amino acids with a short N-terminal cytoplasmic domain (17 amino acids), a hydrophobic transmembrane domain, and a large extracellular domain with nine potential N-linked glycosylation sites (Wu et al. 1990). Topologically, therefore, the BP-1/6C3 antigen resembles NEP and aminopeptidase N. Its possible identity as a metallopeptidase was suggested by the presence of a typical zinc-binding motif (in this case, VVAHELVHQW). The amino acid sequence showed significant homology (36%–38%) with aminopeptidase N, suggesting that it might be another, but related, aminopeptidase. The occurrence of the antigen on renal brush-borders and small intestinal enterocytes further suggests that it might be a member of the brush-border metallopeptidase family listed in Table 1.

In order to test this possibility, Wu et al. (1991) examined which peptidase activity could be depleted from small intestinal brush-border preparations by immunoprecipitation with BP-1/6C3 antisera. The enzyme aminopeptidase A was selectively depleted, and a variety of other evidence confirmed BP-1/6C3 as this particular membrane peptidase. Aminopeptidase A had previously been described as a microvillar aminopeptidase expressing a preference for an acidic amino acid at the N-terminus of a substrate, and the enzyme is usually assayed with derivatives of glutamic acid, for example, Glu-NNap, Glu-NMec. Metal analysis of purified aminopeptidase A revealed the presence of calcium rather than zinc (Danielsen et al. 1980), although this observation will clearly need to be checked in the light of the typical zinc-binding motif discovered at the active site by cloning and sequencing of the protein.

Two forms of aminopeptidase A are known – a membrane-bound form on cell-surfaces and a soluble form present in serum. Their very close similarity suggests that they may represent products of the same gene (Yamada et al. 1988). The soluble form of aminopeptidase A, secreted during pregnancy, may play an important role in controlling blood pressure during pregnancy (Lalu et al. 1984). A major physiological role for aminopeptidase A is the removal of the N-terminal aspartyl residue from angiotensin I or II at various tissue sites, and the enzyme may be co-expressed in the vicinity of angiotensin II receptors. This would be analogous to the coexpression of CALLA in the vicinity of opioid receptors discussed above. It can upregulate aminopeptidase A expression and pre-B-cell proliferation, and treatment with anti-BP-1 can block the proliferative response

(Welch et al. 1990). Intriguingly, IL-7 has an N-terminal acidic residue which might be susceptible to hydrolysis by aminopeptidase A. Wu et al. (1991) have therefore postulated that the coexpression of the IL-7 receptor and aminopeptidase A on pre-B-cells and on IL-7 producing stromal cells may contribute to an intricate regulatory mechanism for cell signaling.

Another cluster differentiation antigen, CD26, which is a marker of a T-cell subset, has also now been identified as an ectoenzyme, in this case, dipeptidyl peptidase IV (DPP-IV; EC 3.4.14.5; Ulmer et al. 1989). In addition to its presence on a T-cell subset (particularly $CD4^+$ helper cells), DPP-IV is also found on a variety of mammalian cells and tissues. It is most abundant on the renal brush-border, intestinal epithelium, and placenta but is also found in the capillary endothelium and in plasma. Cell surface DPP-IV activity among lymphoid cells is associated with the ability of a cell to produce IL-2 (Scholz et al. 1985). DPP-IV is unusual among brush-broder peptidases in being a serine enzyme and is therefore inhibited by di-isopropylfluorophosphate. Its specificity is to release dipeptides from the N-terminus of a susceptible peptide where Pro (or Ala) is the penultimate residue, i.e., it acts as a post-proline cleaving enzyme. A physiological role for the enzyme in mammalian systems has not been established, although substance P, which has the N-terminal sequence Arg-Pro-Lys-Pro, is susceptible to hydrolysis. In insects, frogs, and yeast DPP IV is believed to play a role in the proteolytic processing of precursors of biologically active peptides, for example, the bee venom peptide melittin (Kreil et al. 1980).

Most interest in DPP-IV, however, has focused on its possible roles in the immune system. It has been proposed that DPP-IV is involved in T-cell activation and regulation of T-cell proliferation (Schon et al. 1985). For example, inhibitors or antibodies to DPP-IV suppress mitogen-induced T-cell proliferation and IL-2 production. This has been shown most recently by Flentke et al. (1991), who produced aminoboronic acid analogs of proline which function as specific DPP-IV inhibitors. The compounds Ala-boroPro and Pro-boroPro both have K_i values in the nanomolar range. Low concentrations of Pro-boroPro were shown to inhibit antigen-induced proliferation and IL-2 production in murine T-cell lines but not to inhibit the response of these T-cells to the mitogenic lectin concanavalin A. These data therefore further support a role for DPP-IV in antigen-induced, but not mitogen-induced, activation of T-lymphocytes. In addition, a number of cytokines have Ala-Pro N-terminal sequences which could render them susceptible to hydrolysis by DPP-IV, for example, IL-1β, IL-2, granulocyte-macrophage colony-stimulating factor and erythropoietin. A feedback regulatory cycle analogous to that suggested for IL-7 and aminopeptidase A could therefore operate in the case of DPP-IV.

Conclusions

Several major types of neuropeptide degradative activities are detected on the cell surfaces and in the peripheral fluids of mammals and invertebrates. They include aminopeptidase, carboxypeptidase, dipeptidylaminopeptidase, and NEP (for review see, Leung and Le 1991). More than one enzyme may be involved in each of these classes of enzyme activities. For example, both NEP and ACE show activity as dipeptidylcarboxypeptidases since they cleave the enkephalins at the Gly-Phe bond to yield tripeptide and dipeptide products (Thorsett and Wyvratt 1987). Thus, the mechanism of immunoactive peptide signal molecule deactivation or metabolism may be quite complex.

Enkephalin released by endocrine structures or immunocytes into the peripheral fluid is undoubtedly subjected to the degradative actions of these octoenzymes. The functional role of this degradative action in transit to the target cells is not known at this time. It is unclear why it is necessary to degrade enkephalin, which apparently is on transit from one location of the body to another, unless it has multifocal targets, suggesting that there exists a mechanism to protect it from these potential lethal attacks until it reaches a particular locus of action. There appears to be an endogenous mechanism which protects enkephalins during their travel in the various fluids. This type of protective mechanism has been suggested by Marini et al. (1990). It remains to be determined whether a similar protective mechanism is also present in invertebrate hemolymph. Preliminary studies indicate that this may be the case (Stefano, unpublished).

The study of invertebrate hemolymph instead of serum as an experimental model offers two important advantages. First, hemolymph is less complex than serum in its composition. The amount of lipids and proteins present in serum is far greater than that in hemolymph. Since the degradation of enkephalin in mammalian serum and hemolymph of some invertebrates is similar, the simpler composition of hemolymph provides an advantage in the purification of enzymes and the interpretation of experimental data. Second, data obtained from hemolymph also give important information on the evolution of the immune/defense system. Thus, it may prove to be strategically expedient first to derive a working model from hemolymph and then to expand it to the more complex mammalian system.

There is sufficient evidence at present to indicate that these enzymes in mammals and invertebrates are similar in nature and are evolutionarily related (Shipp et al. 1990). Neuropeptides which were once thought to be used only in the neuroendocrine system have now been shown to be used for communication in other systems (Smith and Blalock, 1981; Lygren et al. 1984).

The fact that respective enzyme inhibitors can potentiate a Met-enkephalin mediated response both in vivo and in vitro strongly suggests that endogenous Met-enkephalin is important as an immunoregulatory and autoimmunoregulatory substance. This is further strengthened by the fact that there appear to be several mechanisms that can terminate its actions as well as reduce its effective concentration. From this we can surmise that enkephalins and possibly other signal molecules are shielded until "conditions" are right. Again, the fact that the mechanisms discussed exist in animals separated by 500 million years of evolution underscores the significance of Met-enkephalin in neuroimmunoregulatory processes.

Finally, several mammalian cluster differentiation antigens have a double identity:CALLA/CD10 for example, serves as tumor marker. It is likely that further differentiation antigens will be associated with other ectoenzyme activities. Study of such enzymatic activities in invertebrates may well throw light on their function in higher organisms including the human.

References

Barnes K, Turner AJ, Kenny AJ (1988) Electronmicroscopic immunocytochemistry of pig brain shows that endopeptidase-24.11 is localized in neuronal membranes. Neurosci Lett 94:64–69

Bowes MA, Kenny AJ (1986) Endopeptidase-24.11 in pig lymph nodes: purification and immunocytochemical identification in reticular cells. Biochem J 236:801–810

Brown G, Hogg N, Greaves M (1975) Candidate leukemia-specific antigen in man. Nature 258:454–456

Burstein Y, Buchner V, Pecht M, Trainin N (1988) Thymic humoral factor gamma2: purification and amino acid sequence of an immunoregulatory peptide from calf thymus. Biochemistry 27:4066–4071

Carrel S, De Tribolet N, Gross N (1982) Expression of HLA-DR and common acute lymphoblastic leukemia antigens on glioma cells. Eur J Immunol 23:354–357

Carrel S, Schmidt-Kessen A, Mach J-P, Heumann D, Girardet C (1983) Expression of common acute lymphoblastic leukemia antigen (CALLA) on human malignant melanoma cell lines. J Immunol 130:2456–2466

Coletti-Previero MA, Mattras H, Descomps B, Previero A (1981) Purification and substrate characterization of a human enkephalin-degrading aminopeptidase. Biochem Biophys Acta 657:122–127

Cooper MD, Mulvaney D, Continho A, Cazenave P (1986) A novel cell surface molecule on early B-lineage cells. Nature 321:616–618

Danielsen AM, Noren O, Sjostrom H, Ingram J, Kenny AJ (1980) Aspartate aminopeptidase: purification by immunoadsorbent chromatography and properties of the detergent and proteinase-solubilized forms. Biochem J 189:591–603

Devault A, Lazure C, Nault C, LeMoual H, Seidah NG, Chretien M, Kahn P, Powell J, Mallet J, Beaumont A, Roques BP, Crine P, Boileau G (1987) Amino acid sequence of rabbit kidney neutral endopeptidase 24.11 (enkephalinase) deduced from a complementary DNA. EMBO J 6:1317–1322

Dupont A, Cusan L, Garon M, Alvarado-Urbina G, Labrie F (1977) Extremely rapid degradation of [^{3}H]-methionine-enkephalin by various rat tissues in vivo and in vitro. Life Sci 21:907–914

Erdös EG, Wagner B, Harburg CB, Painter RG, Skidgel RA, Fa X (1989) Down-regulation and inactivation of neutral endopeptidase 24.11 (enkephalinase) in human neutrophils. J Biol Chem 264:14519–14523

Fischer EG, Falke NE (1987) Interaction of met-enkephalin with human granulocytes. Ann NY Acad Sci 496:146–150

Flentke GR, Munoz E, Huber BT, Plant AG, Kettner CA, Bachovchin WW (1991) Inhibition of dipeptidylaminopeptidase IV (DP-IV) by Xoa-boroPro dipeptides and use of these inhibitors to examine the role of DP-IV in T cell formation. Proc Natl Acad Sci USA 88:1556-1559

Fulcher IS, Pappin DJC, Kenny AJ (1986) The N-terminal amino acid sequence of pig kidney endopeptidase-24.11 shows homology with pro-sucrase-isomaltase. Biochem J 240:305–308

Funkhouser JD, Tangada SD, Jones M, O SJ, Peterson DA (1991) p146 type II alveolar epithelial cell antigen is identical to aminopeptidase N. Am J Physiol 260:274–279

Gee NS, Bowes MA, Buck P, Kenny AJ (1985) An immunoradiometric assay for endopeptidase-24.11 shows it to be a widely distributed enzyme in pig tissues. Biochem J 228:119–126

Greaves MF, Brown G, Rapson N, Lister TA (1975) Antisera to acute lymphoblastic leukemia cells. Clin Immunol Immunopathol 4:67–72

Greaves MF, Hairi G, Newman RA, Sutherland DR, Ritter MA, Ritz J (1983) Selective expression of the common acute lymphoblastic leukemia (gp100) antigen on immature lymphoid cells and their malignant counterparts. Blood 61:628–639

Hambrook JM, Morgan BA, Rance MJ, Smith CFC (1976) Mode of deactivation of the enkephalins by rat and human plasma and rat brain homogenates. Nature 262:782–783

Hersh LB, Morihara K (1986) Comparison of the subsite specificity of the mammalian neutral endopeptidase-24.11 (enkephalinase) to the bacterial neutral endopeptidase thermolysin. J Biol Chem 261:6433–6437

Hioki Y, Okada K, Ito H, Matsuyama K, Yano M (1991) Endothelin converting enzyme of bovine carotid artery smooth muscle cells. Biochem Biophys Res Commun 174:446–451

Hussain MM, Tranum-Jensen J, Noren O, Sjostrom H, Christiansen K (1981) Reconstitution of purified amphiphilic pig intestinal microvillus aminopeptidase. Biochem J 199:179–186

Indig FE, Pecht M, Trainin N, Burstein Y, Blumberg S (1991) Hydrolysis of thymic humoral factor gamma 2 by neutral endopeptidase EC 3.4.24.11 Biochem J 278:891–894

Isaac RE (1988) Neuropeptide-degrading endopeptidase activity of locust (Schistocerca gregaria) synaptic membranes. Biochem J 255:843–847

Jongeneel CV, Bouvier J, Bairoch A (1989) A unique signature identifies a family of zinc-dependent metallopeptidases. FEBS Lett 242:211–214

Kenny AL, Turner AJ (eds) (1987) Mammalian ectoenzymes, Elsevier, Amsterdam

Kenny AJ, Stephenson SL, Turner AJ (1987) Cell-surface peptidases. In: Kenny AJ, Turner AJ (eds) Mammalian ectoenzymes. Elsevier, Amsterdam, pp 169–210

Kerr MA, Kenny AJ (1974) The purification and specificities of a neutral endopeptidase from rabbit kidney brush border. Biochem J 137:477–488

Kreil G, Haiml L, Suchanek G (1980) Stepwise cleavage of the pro part of promelittin by dipeptidyl peptidase IV. Evidence for a new type type of precursor-product conversion. Eur J Biochem 111:49–58

Lalu K, Lameplo S, Nummelin-Kortelainen M, Vanha-Perttula T (1984) Purification and partial characterization of aminopeptidase A from the serum of pregnant and non-pregnant women, Biochim Biophys Acta 789:324–333

Lane A, Rance MJ, Walter DS (1977) Subcellular localization of leucine-enkephalin hydrolyzing activity in rat brain. Nature 269:75–76

LeTarte M, Vera S, Tran R, Addis JB, Omizuka RJ, Quackenbush EJ, Jongeneel CV, McInnes RR (1988) Common acute lymphocytic leukemia antigen is identical to neutral endopeptidase. J Exp Med 168:1247–1253

Leung MK (1990) Degradation of opioid peptides in invertebrate hemolymph. International workshop on developmental and comparative neuroimmunology, abstract no 12

Leung MK, Le SX (1991) Enkephalin degradative enzymes in serum and hemolymph: a comparative study. Adv. Neuroimmunol 1:17–26

Leung MK, Lundy J (1990) Opioid neuropeptides in invertebrate haemolymph. In: Forey E, Stefano GB (eds) Comparative aspects of neuropeptides. Manchester University Press, Manchester, pp 516–517

Look AT, Ashmun RA, Shapiro LH, Peiper SE (1989) Human myeloid plasma membrane glycoprotein CD13 (gp150) is identical to aminopeptidase. N. J Clin Invest 83:1299–1307

Lygren J, Revhaug PG, Burhol KE, Giercksky KE, Jenssen TG (1984) Vasoactive intestinal peptide and somatostatin in leukocytes. Scand J Clin Lab Invest 44:347–351

Malfroy B, Swertz JB, Guyon A, Roques BP, Schwartz JC (1978) High affinity enkephalin-degrading peptidase in brain is increased after morphine. Nature 276:523–526

Malfroy B, Schofield P, Kuang WJ, Seeburg PH, Mason AJ, Henzel WJ (1987) Molecular cloning and amino acid sequence of rat enkephalinase. Biochem Biophys Res Commun 144:59–66

Malfroy B, Kuang WJ, Seeburg PH, Mason AJ, Schofield PR (1988) Molecular cloning and amino acid sequence of human enkephalinase (neutral endopeptidase). FEBS Lett 229:206–210

Marini M, Roscetti G, Bongiorno L, Urbani A, Roda LG (1990) Hydrolysis and protection from hydrolysis of enkephalins in human plasma. Neurochem Res 15:61–67

Massoulie J, Bon S (1982) The molecular forms of cholinesterase and acetylcholinesterase in vertebrates. Annu Rev Neurosci 5:57–106

Matsas R, Fulcher IS, Kenny AJ, Turner AJ (1983) Substance P and [Leu] enkephalin are hydrolyzed by an enzyme in pig caudate membranes that is identical with the endopeptidase of kidney microvilli. Proc Natl Acad Sci USA 80:3111–3115

Matsas R, Kenny J, Turner AJ (1984) The metabolism of neuropeptides: the hydrolysis of peptides, including enkephalins, tachykinins and their analogues by endopeptidase-24.11. Biochem J 223:433–440

Matsas R, Stephenson SL, Hryszko J, Kenny AJ, Turner AJ (1985) The metabolism of neuropeptides: phase-separation of synaptic membrane preparations with Triton X-114 reveals the presence of aminopeptidase N. Biochem J 231:445–449

Matsas R, Kenny AJ, Turner AJ (1986) An immunohistochemical study of endopeptidase-24.11 ('enkephalinase') in the pig nervous system. Neuroscience 18:991–1012

Medeiros MS, Balmforth AJ, Vaughan PFT, Turner AJ (1991) Hydrolysis of atrial and brain natriuretic peptides by the human astrocytoma clone D384 and the neuroblastoma line SH-SY5Y. Neuroendocrinology 54:295–302

Meglitsch PA (1967) In: Invertebrate zoology. Oxford University Press, New York

Painter RG, Dukes R, Sullivan J, Carter R, Erdös EG, Johnson AR (1988) Function of neutral endopeptidase on the cell membrane of human neutrophils. J. Biol Chem 263:9456–9461

Peirart ME, Najdovski T, Appelboom TE, Deschodt-Lanckmann MM (1988) Effect of human endopeptidase-24.11 ("enkephalinase") on IL-1-induced thymocyte proliferation activity. J Immunol 140:3808–3811

Poole S, Bird TA, Selkirk S, Gaines-Das RE, Choudry Y, Stephenson SL, Kenny AJ, Saklatvala J (1990) Fate of injected interleukin-1 in rats: sequestration and degradation in kidney. Cytokine 2:416–422

Raftery MA, Hunkapillar MW, Strader CD, Hood LE (1980) Acetylcholine receptor: complex of homologous subunits. Science 208:1454–1457

Ritz J, Pesando JM, Notis-McConarty J, Lazarus H, Schlossman SF (1980) A monoclonal antibody to human acute lymphoblastic leukemia antigen. Nature 283:583–585

Roques BP, Beaumont A (1990) Neutral endopeptidase-24.11 inhibitors: from analgesics to antihypertensives. Trends Pharmacol Sci 11: 245–249

Scholz W, Mentlein R, Heymann E, Feller AC, Flad HD (1985) Interleukin-2 production by human T lymphocytes identified by antibodies to dipeptidyl peptidase IV. Cell Immunol 89:11–19

Schon E, Mansfeld HW, Demuth HU, Barth A, Ansorge S (1985) The dipeptidyl peptidase IV, a membrane enzyme involved in the proliferation of T lymphocytes. Biomed Biochim Acta 44:K9–K15

Shipp MA, Richardson NE, Sayre PH, Brown NR, Masteller EL, Clayton LK, Ritz J, Reinherz EL (1988) Molecular cloning of the common acute lymphoblastic leukemia antigen (CALLA) identifies a type II integral membrane protein. Proc Natl Acad Sci USA 85:4819–4823

Shipp MA, Vijayaraghavan J, Schmidt EV, Masteller EL, D'Adamio L, Hersh LB, Reinherz EL (1989) Common acute lymphoblastic leukemia antigen (CALLA) is active neutral endopeptidase 24.11 ("enkephalinase"):direct evidence by cDNA transfection analysis. Proc Natl Acad Sci USA 86:297–301

Shipp MA, Stefano GB, D'Adamio L, Switzer SN, Howard FD, Sinisterra J, Scharrer B, Reinherz EL (1990) Down-regulation of enkephalin mediated inflammatory responses by CD10/neutral endopeptidase 24.11. Nature 347:394–396

Smith EM, Blalock JE (1981) Human lymphocyte production of ACTH and endorphin-like substances: associated with leukocyte interferon. Proc Natl Acad Sci USA 78:7530–7534

Stefano GB, Leung MK, Zhao X, Scharrer B (1989a) Evidence for the involvement of opioid neuropeptides in the adherence and migration of immunocompetent invertebrate hemocytes. Proc Natl Acad Sci USA 86:626–630

Stefano GB, Cadet P, Scharrer B (1989b) Stimulatory effects of opioid neuropeptides on locomotory activity and conformational changes in invertebrate and human immunocytes: evidence for a subtype of opioid receptor. Proc Natl Acad Sci USA 86:6307–6311

Stefano GB, Shipp MA, Scharrer B (1991) A possible immunoregulatory function for Met-enkephalin-Arg6-Phe7 involving human and invertebrate granulocytes. J Neuroimmunol 31: 97–103

Stephenson SL, Kenny AJ (1987) The hydrolysis of human atrial natriuretic peptide by pig kidney microvillar membranes is initiated by endopeptidase-24.11. Biochem J 243:183–187

Thorsett ED, Wyvratt MJ (1987) Inhibition of zinc peptidases that hydrolyse neuropeptides. In: Turner AJ (ed) Neuropeptides and their peptidases. VCH, New York, pp 229–292

Tredosiewicz LK, Malizia G, Oakes J, Losowsky M, Janossy G (1985) Expression of the common acute lymphoblastic leukemia antigen (CALLA, gp100) in the brush border of normal jejunum and jejunum of patients with coeliac disease. J Clin Pathol 38:1002–1006

Turner AJ (ed) (1987) Neuropeptides and their peptidases. Ellis Horwood, Chichester

Turner AJ, Dowdall MJ (1984) The metabolism of neuropeptides: both phosphoramidon-sensitive and captopril–sensitive metallopeptidases are present in the electric organ of Torpedo marmorata. Biochem J 222:255–259

Turner AJ, Matsas R, Kenny AJ (1985) Are there neuropeptide-specific peptidases? Biochem Pharmacol 34:1347–1356

Turner AJ, Hooper NM, Kenny AJ (1987) Neuropeptide metabolism. In: Kenny AJ, Turner AJ (eds) Mammalian ectoenzymes. Elsevier, Amsterdam, 211–248

Ulmer AJ, Mattern T, Feller AC, Heymann E, Flad H-D (1989) TII19–4–7 and 4EL1C7 but not B1.19.2 (all clustered in CDw26) bind to dipeptidyl peptidase IV (DPP-IV). 7th international congress of immunology. Fisher, Stuttgart, p 151 (abstract)

Van Epps DE, Kutvirt SJ (1987) Modulation of human neutrophil adherence by β-endorphin and Met-enkephalin. J Neuroimmunol 15:219–228

Van Epps DE, Saland L (1984) β-endorphin and Met-enkephalin stimulate human peripheral blood mononuclear cell chemotaxis. J Immunol 132:3046–3053

Venturelli F, Roscetti G, Posssenti R, Vita F, Roda LG (1985) Peripheral enkephalin hydrolysis in different animal species: a comparative study. Neurochem Res 10:333–342

Vogel Z, Altstein M (1979) The effect of puromycin on the biological activity of Leu-enkephalin. FEBS Lett 98:44–47

Vogt-Schaden M, Ciagelmann M, Hock D, Herbst F, Forssmann WG (1989) Degradation of porcine brain natriuretic peptide (pBNP-26) by endoprotease-24.11 from kidney cortical membranes. Biochem biophys Res Commun 161:1177–1183

Welch PA, Burrows PD, Gillis S, Cooper MD (1990) J Cell Biochem [Suppl] 14D:267 (abstract)

Wilk S (1986) Neuropeptide-specific peptidases: does brain contain a specific TRH-degrading enzyme? Life Sci 39:1487–1492

Wu Q, Tidmarsh GF, Welch PA, Pierce JH, Weissman IL, Cooper MD (1989) The early B lineage antigen BP-1 and the transformation-associated antigen 6C3 are on the same molecule. J Immunol 143:3303–3308

Wu Q, Lahti JM, Air GM, Burrows PD, Cooper MD (1990) Molecular cloning of the murine BP-1/6C3 antigen: a member of the zinc-dependent metallopeptidase family. Proc Natl Acad Sci USA 87:993–997

Wu Q, Li L, Cooper MD, Pierres M, Gorvel JP (1991) Aminopeptidase A activity of the murine B-lymphocyte differentiation antigen BP-1/6C3. Proc Natl Acad Sci USA 88:676–680

Yamada R, Mizutani S, Kuranchi O, Okono K, Imaizumi H, Narita O, Tomoda Y (1988) Purification and characterization of human placental aminopeptidase A. Enzyme 40:223–230

Subject Index